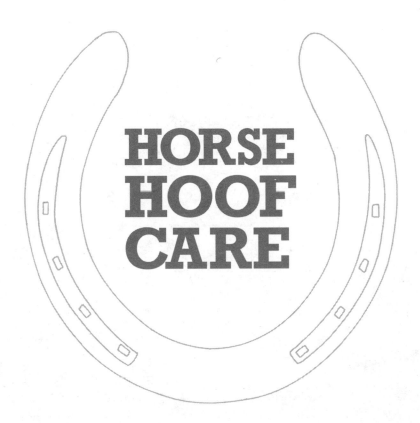

HORSE
HOOF
CARE

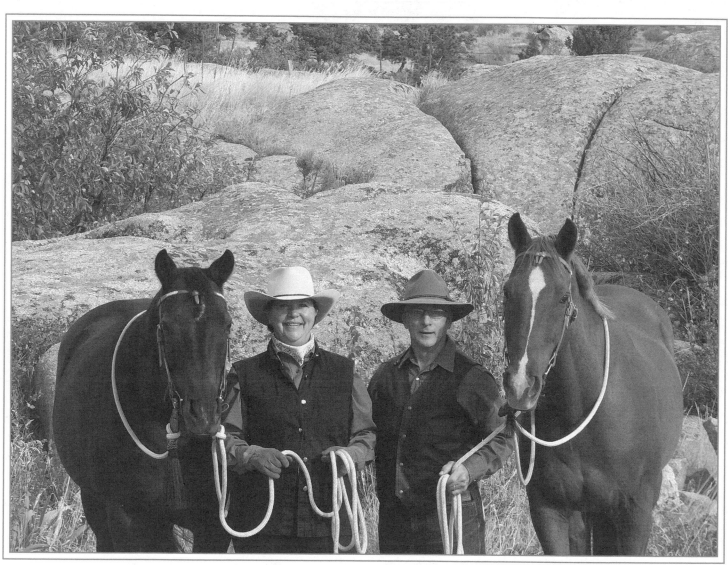

HORSE HOOF CARE

Cherry Hill
and
Richard Klimesh

Photography by Cherry Hill and Richard Klimesh

Illustrations by Richard Klimesh

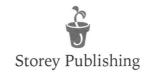

Storey Publishing

The mission of Storey Publishing is to serve our customers by publishing practical information that encourages personal independence in harmony with the environment.

Edited by Deborah Burns and Rebekah Boyd-Owens
Art direction and book design by Cynthia N. McFarland
Cover design by Joseph R. Williams
Text production by Jennifer Jepson Smith

Cover photography by © Cherry Hill
Interior photography by © Cherry Hill and Richard Klimesh
Illustrations by Richard Klimesh
Author photograph by Randy Dunn

Indexed by Susan Olason, Knowledge Maps & Indexes

Printed in the United States by Versa Press
10 9 8 7 6 5 4 3 2 1

Library of Congress Cataloging-in-Publication Data
Hill, Cherry, 1947–
  Horse hoof care / Cherry Hill and Richard Klimesh.
      p. cm.
  Includes bibliographical references and index.
  ISBN 978-1-60342-088-4 (pbk. : alk. paper)
  1. Hoofs—Care and hygiene. 2. Horses—Health.
  I. Klimesh, Richard. II. Title.
SF907.H53 2009
636.1'0897585—dc22
                                        2008032435

CONTENTS

Notes from the Authors vi

1 HOOF KNOWLEDGE 1
Hoof Parts and Function • Hoofology • Hoof Growth
and Shape • Hoof Care Hokum

2 PROFESSIONAL HELPERS 9
Why You Need a Farrier • What Makes a Good Far-
rier? • Finding a Farrier • Why You Need a
Veterinarian • Finding an Equine Veterinarian

3 FACILITIES 14
Keep Them Dry • Stall Flooring • Types of Bedding •
Pen and Pasture • Work Areas • Tying Options

4 TRAINING 22
Early Hoof-Handling Lessons • Picking Up a Horse's
Foot • Working Positions

5 MANAGEMENT 30
A Balanced Diet • Exercise for Strong Hooves •
Clean and Dry Stalls • Daily Hoof Check •
Hoof Cleaning

6 TACK AND TOOLS 40
Halters • Hoof Tools • Hoof Boots • Shoe
Removal Kit

7 BAREFOOT 46
To Shoe or Not to Shoe • Should You Pull Shoes
for Winter? • Bare Facts • Barefoot Trim • Foals,
Weanlings, and Yearlings • Boots for Bare Hooves •
Hoof Boots

8 HORSESHOES, AND WHY 57
Types of Hoof Care • Reasons for Shoeing • Horse-
shoe Anatomy • Shoe Types • Pads • Hoof Packing •
Clips • Traction • Winter Shoeing

9 SHOEING, AND HOW . . . . , 72
Hot or Cold Shoes? • Shoeing Steps • Shaping the
Hoof • Measuring and Balancing • Fitting and Nailing • Finishing • The Horseshoe Nail • New Shoes
or Reset?

10 OWNER SKILLS 81
Know Good Work When You See It • Hoof Angles •
Heel Support • Holding a Horse for the Farrier •
Safe Positioning • Removing a Shoe • Temporary
Hoof Protection • Applying Hoof Products • Hoof
Polish Tips

11 HOOF PROBLEMS AND FIXES 97
Lost Shoes • Hoof Cracks • Crack Treatment •
Thrush Treatment • Long Toe/Low Heel • Con-
tracted Heels • Mismatched Hooves • Stumbling •
Forging and Overreaching • Interfering

12 CALL THE VET 120
Bruises, Abcesses, and Corns • Seedy Toe and White
Line Disease • Clubfoot • Navicular Syndrome •
Laminitis

13 TEAMWORK 136
Your Role • A Working Partnership • Scheduling a
Farrier Visit • Keeping a Good Farrier • Rewards

Glossary 144

Resource Guide 148

Index 150

NOTES FROM THE AUTHORS

WHEN WE THINK OF A HORSE, we think of powerful muscles and athletic motion with mane and tail flowing. We picture a beautiful head and an expressive eye showing a generous, cooperative nature. We see behavior that demonstrates both curiosity and honesty. There is one trait we often take for granted, however: healthy, sound hooves. Without them, the noble horse is often transformed into an uncomfortable, tentative, grouchy, sullen, and tuned-out beast. No foot, no horse.

As a horse-show judge and riding instructor for many years, I have seen many fat and shiny overgroomed horses carrying thousands of dollars' worth of tack and rider attire, dragging themselves around the ring with the most neglected hooves imaginable. Right there in the show arena or lesson ring, I've seen too many hooves with extremely long toes and low heels, quarters that have overgrown the shoes, and cracks galore. I've heard loose shoes rattling; seen mincing, wincing travel; and pulled many a lame horse out of a class, hoping the owner or rider would then take heed of the horse's hoof-care needs.

Sadly, hoof care and horseshoeing are two topics that many horse owners seem to know very little about. Only when a horse develops a debilitating lameness do hooves suddenly become a topic of interest. Like many aspects of horse care, however, good management prevents many hoof problems; an ounce of prevention is truly worth a pound of cure.

Once you learn a few basic hoof-care skills and get in the habit of cleaning hooves, feeding for hoof quality, and scheduling regular farrier care, your horse will benefit greatly. And in the long run, it will save you time and money.

Your horse and I thank you for picking up this book. You're obviously one of those horse owners who cares about your horse's comfort and soundness or you wouldn't have read this far, so I applaud your dedication! I hope that the hoof-care information Richard and I share with you in this book will help you to help your horse be the best he can be — healthy, sound, and full of life.

Cherry Hill

THIRTY YEARS AGO, when I was an eager farrier-science grad beginning my career, the choice of resources for farriers was limited, to say the least. Good-quality horseshoes were hard to find, and many farriers forged the shoes they used. Horseshoe nails were thick and tended to split the hoof. Hoof-repair materials consisted mainly of auto body filler and fiberglass, which worked well on cars and boats but not very well on hooves. Hoof boots were a novelty then, and they were cumbersome to apply and difficult to keep on. Clinics and workshops were few and far between, and there were no online forums because, of course, there was no Internet.

Over the years, several varieties of well-designed keg shoes became available. Coupled with the slimmer nails that I had been hoping for, these improved shoes made my job more efficient and less damaging to hooves. Hoof sealers were developed that actually improved hoof quality, and new hoof-repair materials not only stuck to the hoof but also mimicked the characteristics of a hoof, which allowed a farrier to trim and nail into repaired areas as the hoof grew. Today, we have glue-on shoes that often stay affixed better than nailed shoes and that are especially helpful with very young or lame horses. A wide variety of modern high-quality hoof boots now enable many horses to be ridden in comfort yet be barefoot during their off time.

Ongoing research has disproved established beliefs about hoof care and has led to new, successful treatments for what were once thought to be commonly fatal hoof diseases, specifically laminitis and navicular syndrome. The World Wide Web increases farrier and horse-owner access to much of this research and lets them exchange opinions and advice.

What hasn't changed is the fact that a domestic horse still relies totally on his owner for all the things necessary for growing and maintaining strong healthy hooves. The key ingredients for great hooves are simple, and they begin with commitment and regular care. I hope this book will give you incentive to design an effective hoof-care plan that will enable you and your equine partner to enjoy many happy years together.

Richard Klimesh

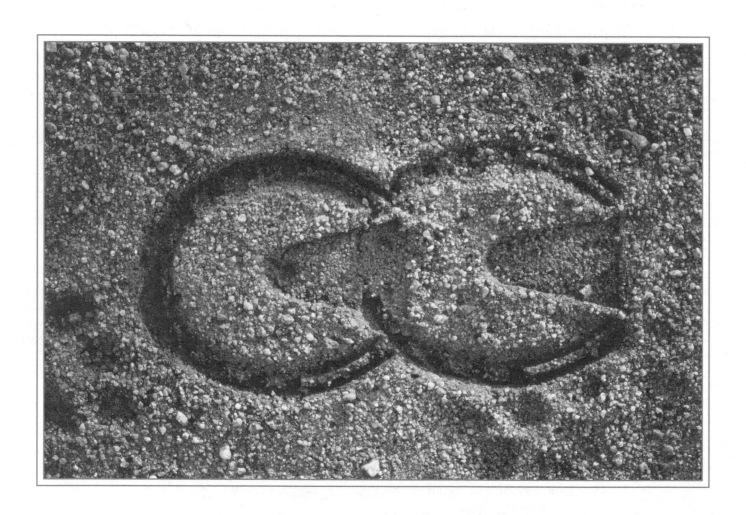

-1-
HOOF KNOWLEDGE

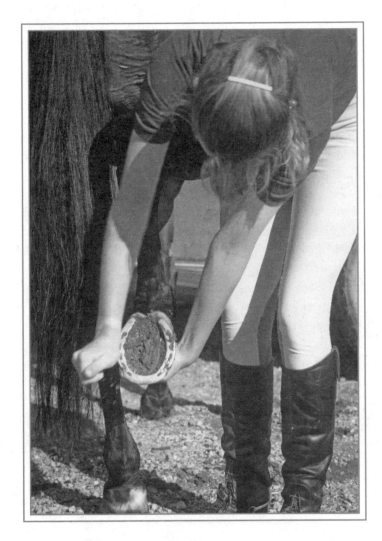

Why do some horses move boldly and confidently while others move meekly and cautiously? Why do some horses develop and maintain solid, healthy hooves while others' hooves become small and contracted? What makes some hooves tough and durable and others brittle and pithy?

The quality and health of a hoof depend on genetics and environment. A horse inherits the potential for good or poor hooves from his parents. Environmental factors that influence hoof health include nutrition, sanitation, moisture, and exercise. As director of your horse's hoof health management program, a good place to start is with a basic knowledge of how the foot works.

FOOT OR HOOF?

Although the terms "hoof" and "foot" are used interchangeably in conversation, "hoof" more specifically refers to the tough, horny external material making up the hoof wall, sole, and frog. "Foot" refers to the hoof and all of its internal parts including bones, tendons, ligaments, nerves, and blood vessels.

HOOF PARTS AND FUNCTION

Knowing the names of basic foot parts will allow you to communicate more effectively with your farrier and veterinarian.

The Bottom of a Hoof

The bottom of the hoof is divided into three general sections: the toe, the quarters, and the heels. The parts of the hoof that you can see — the hoof wall, frog, and sole — are all insensitive, much like your fingernails.

Sensitive hoof tissues contain blood vessels and nerves. When sensitive tissues are injured, they will bleed and cause the horse pain.

Insensitive hoof tissues do not contain blood vessels or nerves. They can withstand wear and tear, trimming, rasping, and nailing without bleeding or causing the horse pain.

1

Inside a Hoof

The **white line** is an important junction: it indicates where the sole meets the hoof wall. It is also the place where insensitive laminae attached to the hoof wall connect with sensitive laminae attached to the coffin bone.

The **bars** are portions of the hoof wall that angle forward from the buttress at the heels along each side of the frog.

The **sole** is the hard material covering most of the bottom of the hoof. A well-conformed sole is cupped; this concave shape keeps it from touching hard flat ground and allows the sole to descend as the foot bears weight.

The **frog** is a rubberlike V-shaped cushion located between the heels. It provides traction with the ground and protects the sensitive inner structures of the hoof while allowing the hoof capsule to expand and contract as the hoof bears weight.

Deep grooves along each side of the frog, called **collateral clefts** or **sulci**, separate the frog from the bars and sole.

The **central cleft**, or **central sulcus**, marks the centerline of the frog.

The **heel bulbs** are a rounded area at the back of the hoof where the frog merges with the skin of the foot.

A cross-section of the hoof reveals:

The **coronary band (coronet)** is a soft ridge around the top of the hoof that produces hoof growth. The hoof wall grows from the coronary band much as your fingernail grows from your cuticle.

The **periople** and **stratum tectorum** make up a thin outer covering that protects the hoof. It is thickest just below the coronary band.

The bulk of the hoof wall, the **hoof horn**, is made up of tightly packed parallel bundles of horn tubules.

The lowest bone in the hoof is shaped like the hoof and has many names: **coffin bone**, **pedal bone**, **distal phalanx**, **third phalanx**, **PIII**, and **P3**.

The **navicular bone** is located behind the coffin bone.

Leaves of insensitive **laminae** on the inside of the hoof wall interlock with sensitive laminae on the surface of the coffin bone. The coffin bone is suspended more by the laminae above it than supported from below by the sole and the frog.

A **flexor tendon** runs down the back of the leg between the sesamoid bones and over the navicular bone and attaches to the bottom of the coffin bone. It lifts the foot and hinges it backward.

An **extensor tendon** runs down the front of the leg and attaches to the top of the coffin bone. It hinges the foot forward to position the hoof for landing.

Hoof Bottom

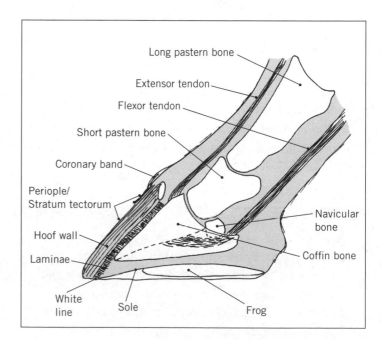

Hoof Cross-Section

H O O F O L O G Y

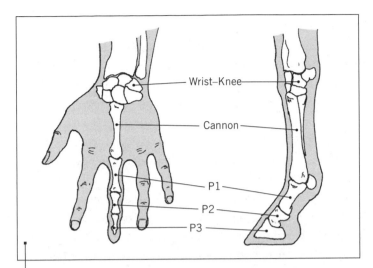

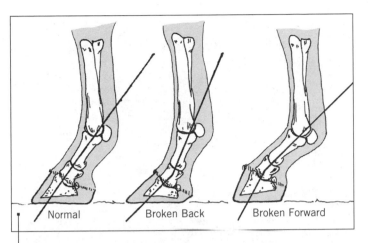

Human Hand and Horse Foot Compared

The **coffin bone (P3)** corresponds to the end bone in your finger.

The **short pastern bone** (also called the **second phalanx** or **P2**) forms a joint with the coffin bone and the navicular bone. It corresponds to the middle bone in your finger.

The **long pastern bone** (also called the **first phalanx** or **P1**) forms a joint with the short pastern bone at the pastern, just above the coronet. The long pastern bone corresponds to the longest bone in your finger.

The **cannon bone** corresponds to the long central bone in your hand.

The horse's **knee** corresponds to your wrist, his **hock** to your ankle.

Hoof and Pastern Angle

Hoof angle is the angle between the front surface of the hoof and the ground when the horse is standing on a flat surface. When a hoof is in balance, an imaginary line through the center of the long pastern bone will be parallel to the front of the coffin bone. In a normal hoof, this line will also be parallel to the front of the hoof wall. Normal hoof angles range from 52 to 60 degrees. Hoof-angle imbalance can lead to all sorts of problems, including permanent lameness. A hoof angle is said to be "broken back" when the toe is too long and the heels are too low. This is the most common and most serious hoof imbalance. A hoof angle is "broken forward" when the heels are too high and the toe is too short.

Coffin Bone Angle

In a healthy, balanced foot, the front of the coffin bone is parallel to the front of the hoof wall, while the bottom of the coffin bone angles up at the back 2 to 3 degrees from the horizontal plane. Because we can't see the coffin bone, we rely on hoof angle, measured by a hoof protractor or by an experienced eye, to align the coffin bone.

On the other hand, when a hoof wall has a dish, bulge, or other distortion or a separation of the laminae, the hoof angle will not match the angle of the hidden coffin bone. The only way to positively determine coffin bone angle, and to assure proper balance, is to take an x-ray of the foot.

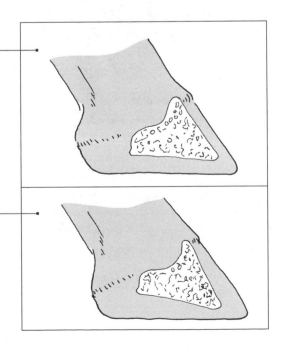

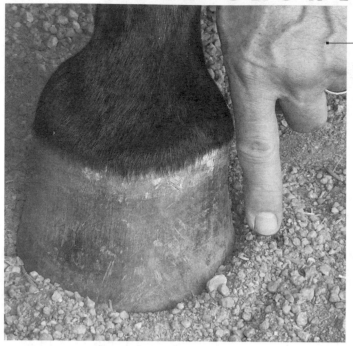

Hoof Growth Rate

Depending on a horse's genetics, diet, exercise, the environment in which he lives, and the season, a hoof can grow immeasurably, or up to ½ inch (1.3 cm) per month, about twice as much as your fingernail. The average growth rate is ¼ inch (0.6 cm) per month. A healthy hoof on a riding horse is approximately 3¼ inches to 3½ inches (8.3–8.9 cm) long at the toe. It can take more than a year for a horse to grow a completely new hoof.

Hoof growth slows during the winter months and increases in the spring and summer. Regular exercise increases blood flow in a horse's feet and makes hooves grow faster. Increased pressure on a portion of the hoof will make that part grow more slowly; that's why a horse with low, overloaded heels will have slower growth at the heels.

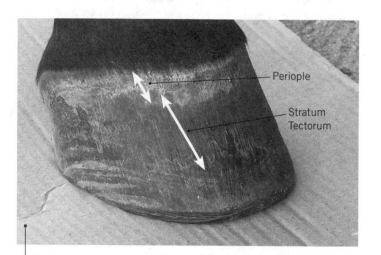

Periople

Stratum
Tectorum

Periople and Stratum Tectorum

The periople is a narrow strip below the coronary band that is like your cuticle. It produces a waxy protective coating that ideally migrates down the hoof and forms a protective layer (the stratum tectorum) that helps maintain moisture balance in the hoof. You can see the stratum tectorum on this hoof as a jagged edge that has migrated two-thirds of the way down the hoof. It often wears away from the lower portion of the hoof.

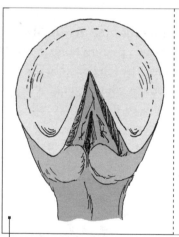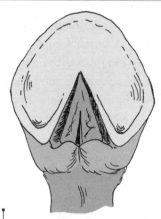

Front Hoof Shape

The front hooves normally carry 65 percent of the horse's (and rider's) weight when at rest and, viewed from the bottom, generally tend to be round in shape. Just like human feet, however, horse feet vary widely in size and shape.

Hind Hoof Shape

Hind hooves are more pointed at the front than fore hooves and are the main source of propulsion for the horse. At rest, the hinds normally carry 35 percent of a horse's weight, but when ridden, a horse can be trained to carry more weight rearward to have a lighter and more agile front end.

A normal healthy hoof should be relatively wide at the heels to transfer concussion and support the horse's weight. If a hoof is imbalanced because of a long toe, or if the hoof is not bearing weight because of lameness, the heels can contract and bind up the foot, resulting in pain to the horse.

You can check for contracted heels using this method of measurement:

1. Measure the width across the heels ¼ inch (0.6 cm) in front of the rearmost point of the buttresses.
2. Then measure the width across the toe 1 inch (2.5 cm) back from the front of the hoof.
3. Compare the measurements. If the heel measurement is less than the toe measurement, the heels are contracted.

If a hoof fits this definition of contracted heels but is balanced due to other criteria, and the animal is sound, there is likely no cause for concern.

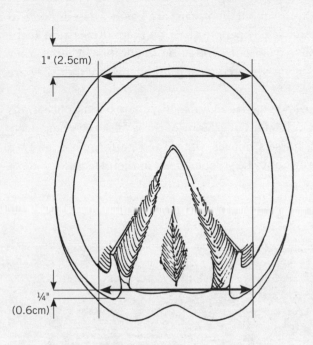

1" (2.5cm)

¼" (0.6cm)

A Hoof Is Like a Cone

A horse's hoof has evolved to be cone shaped: wider at the bottom than at the coronet, with a hoof wall that is straight. In this case straight does not mean vertical, it means a true line from the coronary band to the ground, without dips or bulges.

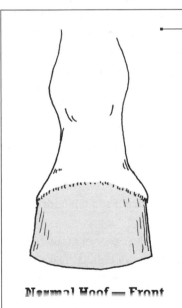

Normal Hoof — Front

Flared Hoof

A hoof wall that is not true but that curves and flares outward at the bottom is much weaker than a straight wall. A flare at the front of a hoof is called a dish. Flares and dishes can lead to many hoof problems, including cracks, broken walls, seedy toe, and lost shoes. Once you know what you are looking for, it is easy to tell if a hoof wall is true or flared.

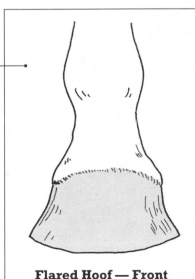

Flared Hoof — Front

HOOF CARE HOKUM

Old notions about hoof care are easily passed along as facts because few people question them. Repetition keeps ideas alive from one generation to another, whether they are based on research or anecdote, and whether they are true or false.

Horseshoeing has an unhealthy share of misconceptions that we call false tales. Many of these false tales negatively affect a horse's hooves, limbs, and performance, and we feel they should be stopped dead in their tracks!

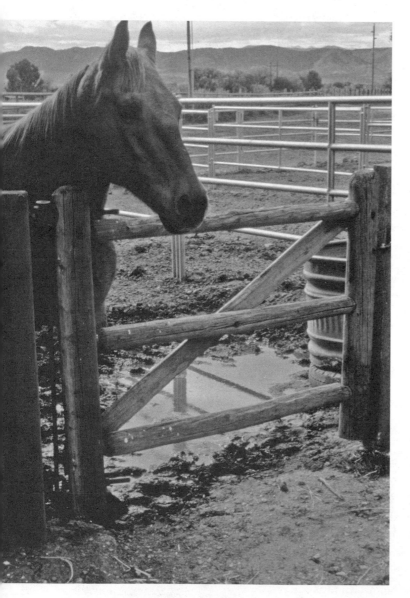

Keep your horse out of the mud and muck.

False Tales

Each of the following false tales is followed by the facts as we know them.

FALSE TALE: *It's good to make a horse stand in water or mud in order to keep his hooves soft.*
FACT: Excess moisture softens and weakens the hoof and makes it more susceptible to bruising, excessive wear, deterioration, and infection. Forcing a horse to stand in mud is rarely a good idea.

FALSE TALE: *Hooves should be trimmed to the ideal angle of 45 degrees.*
FACT: Do you want to hear your farrier laugh? Just ask him when he last saw a 45-degree hoof on a sound horse. Although some books and folklore have touted 45 degrees as the ideal, the angles of normal, healthy hooves are closer to 55 degrees.

FALSE TALE: *A long toe lengthens a horse's stride and makes him softer to ride.*
FACT: In the past, racehorses, hunters, Western pleasure horses, and even reining horses have been shod with long toes, supposedly to gain a performance advantage. Research has proven that long toes do not increase a horse's stride. What they do increase is the likelihood of navicular problems, tendon injuries, and other problems.

FALSE TALE: *A hoof with cracks is too dry.*
FACT: In most cases, hoof cracks indicate just the opposite: the hoof has been too wet!

FALSE TALE: *Hoof dressing adds nutrients to the hoof wall, thereby improving hoof quality.*
FACT: The hoof grows down from the coronet at the top, much as your fingernail grows from the cuticle. The outer hoof wall that you see is essentially dead tissue and cannot utilize any nutrients from hoof dressing. For good-quality hooves, it's more important to see that hoof moisture balance is maintained through exercise and hoof sealers.

FALSE TALE: *Black hooves are better than white hooves.*
FACT: Although many horse owners believe that black hooves are better, research has shown there is no difference in hardness, toughness, or brittleness between white and black hooves.

FALSE TALE: The frog must touch the ground in order for the blood to circulate in the hoof properly.

FACT: The frog has been called an "extra heart" or "blood pump," but it does not have to touch the ground for the hoof to function properly. In fact, a horseshoe typically prevents the frog from coming in contact with the ground, yet many horses that have been shod for decades have sound, healthy feet.

FALSE TALE: Horses that aren't ridden frequently don't need to be trimmed or shod as often as horses that are.

FACT: Whether a horse is ridden or not, his hooves continue to grow, and that is what dictates the need for trimming and reshoeing.

FALSE TALE: Hooves should be trimmed so that they point straight ahead.

FACT: Like people, horses come in all shapes, sizes, and body styles. If a horse's legs are such that his hooves point in (pigeon-toed) or point out (splay-footed), it is generally not a good idea to force them to "look pretty" or to try to fool horse-show judges. In fact, trying to straighten crooked feet and legs can make a sound horse lame. A horse with front feet that toe in will often "paddle" or "wing out" to some extent when he travels; that is, his feet will swing in an arc away from his body and then come back under him to land. This may look comical but seldom causes problems.

It is normal for a horse's hind feet to toe out to some degree. This aids in his natural movement and helps him avoid hitting himself when all legs are in motion. But a horse that toes out on the fronts can have a tendency to swing his feet inward as he travels and hit his opposite leg, sometimes causing injury. Corrective trimming and shoeing can alter movement to avoid interference without compromising soundness.

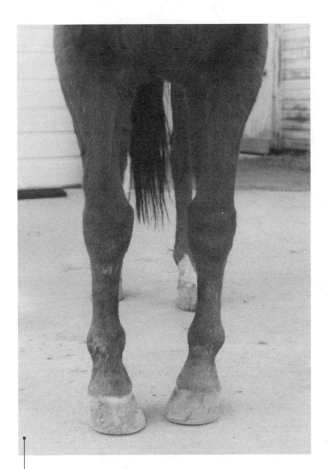

Toes In
It's generally not a good idea to try to force toed-in hooves to be what they are not.

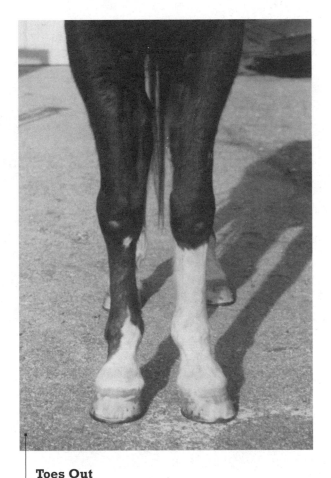

Toes Out
Some toed-out movement is normal, but you and your farrier should evaluate the horse's conformation to decide if corrective treatment is needed.

FALSE TALE: All horses should be allowed to go barefoot for part of the year.

FACT: A healthy hoof that is properly shod does not need to go barefoot. Routinely pulling shoes for the winter can be very harmful to some hooves that require shoes for protection and support. These hooves can be broken and damaged in minutes, and it can take several shoeing periods to restore them to their previous condition. Given proper management, some hooves can maintain soundness without shoes, but they still require regular trimming.

FALSE TALE: Mud will suck a horseshoe right off a hoof.

FACT: This is highly improbable. If you have ever tried to remove a properly applied shoe without first opening the clinches, you know the tremendous amount of force that mud would have to exert to suck off a shoe.

FALSE TALE: The best shoeing job is the one that stays on the longest.

FACT: In fact, the best shoeing job may be the one that comes off easily! Shoes that are fit very close and nailed too securely to the foot can compromise the long-term health of the hoof.

FALSE TALE: Shoeing is a necessary evil.

FACT: This one exasperates a conscientious farrier every time he reads or hears it because the word "evil" implies bad intent. Good shoeing can be one of the kindest gifts you offer your horse. Not only will it not damage his feet, but it could also make him more comfortable and increase his useful life.

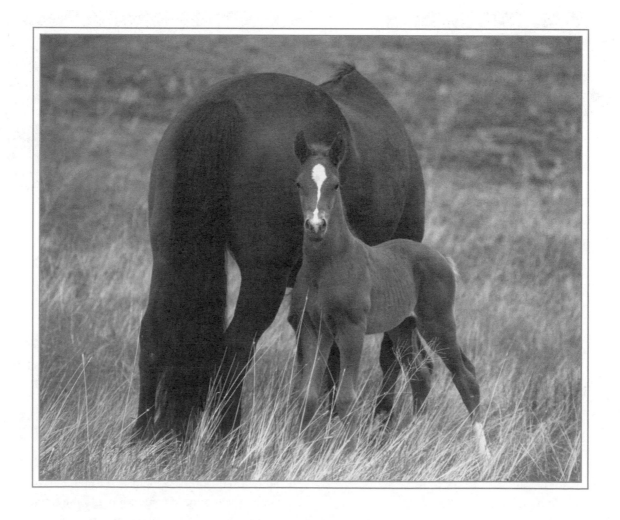

-2-
PROFESSIONAL
HELPERS

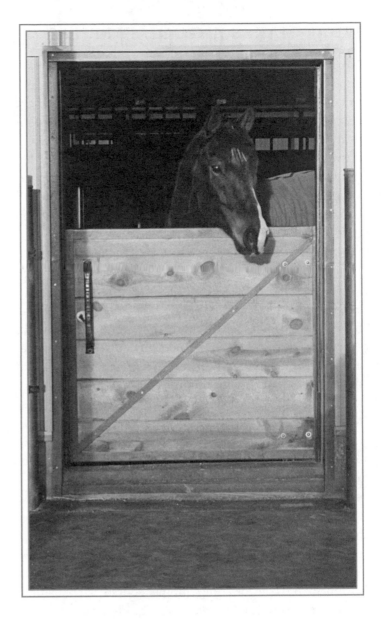

Your horse depends on you to provide food, shelter, exercise, and grooming. You can handle most of those things with little or no help from others. But when it comes to health care and hoof care, it's best if you have reliable professionals on hand to offer guidance and expertise.

"No hoof, no horse" is a saying that is as old as the domestic horse. It used to be that a horse who became lame found that his days were soon over; he was sold for slaughter. But since nearly all slaughter plants in the United States have closed, and because it is very expensive to have a horse put down and buried or cremated, lame horses frequently are sold to someone else to deal with or are turned out to pasture. Often these horses suffer until they die.

Today, a deeper understanding of hoof ailments along with innovative products and technology make it possible to detect and treat minor problems before they cause debilitating lameness. Farriers and veterinarians help many horses with serious diseases, such as navicular syndrome and laminitis, enjoy long comfortable lives.

WHY YOU NEED A FARRIER

You need a good professional farrier because an untrained person can easily make your horse lame with incorrect trimming or shoeing. You might not think you need to pay much attention to your horse's feet as long as he appears sound and is not limping around his pen. The fact is that horses are very adaptable and can often tolerate poor hoof care for many months or even years without obvious signs of lameness. Unfortunately, by the time the first indications of a problem appear, the horse may be irreparably damaged. A farrier is trained to recognize small problems and prevent them from turning into big problems.

WHAT MAKES A GOOD FARRIER?

Storytelling is not a prerequisite to being a good horse-shoer, but being able to accurately explain hoof-care principles to horse owners is important. You should be able to ask your farrier what thrush is and how best to deal with it and get a thorough, intelligent, and accurate answer. Understandably, he can't teach you everything he has learned, but he should be able to give you a succinct answer to any hoof-care question and then recommend books, articles, or Web sites that further discuss the topics that concern or interest you.

Just as there are all levels of horsemen, there are all levels of practicing horseshoers. You will meet people with knowledge that ranges from the very basic skills of self-taught individuals to that of thoroughly educated, high-tech farriers. Horses with abnormal hooves and those with specific performance requirements need the experience and skill of a top-notch farrier. When an inexperienced horseshoer is faced with quarter cracks, underrun heels, laminitis, or navicular syndrome, he may not know what to do. When this happens, his efforts to solve the problem may make the situation worse. A good farrier is open-minded and motivated to seek out advice when faced with an issue he cannot resolve.

The greater the performance demands are on a horse, the more precise his shoeing must be. A backyard pleasure horse with normal hooves may get along fine with shoes put on by a farrier with very basic (but acceptable) skills. However, when that horse is sliding in the reining pen, turning barrels, negotiating a jumper course, or competing on an endurance ride, his shoeing requirements are more specialized.

There are many ways to successfully trim and shoe a horse. Be wary of a shoer or trimmer that promotes one particular method, disregarding all others. The most highly respected and sought-after shoers approach each horse as an individual animal with unique needs. They may be familiar with many methods but are bound by none.

You tend to get what you pay for in farrier service, as you would when buying a saddle or taking a riding lesson. Today, the cost of standard shoeing (four keg shoes) across the United States can range from $45 to $180, a trimming from $25 to $60. Prices vary regionally, and within a region the variation in prices will be based on a farrier's level of experience, education, skill, demand, and location.

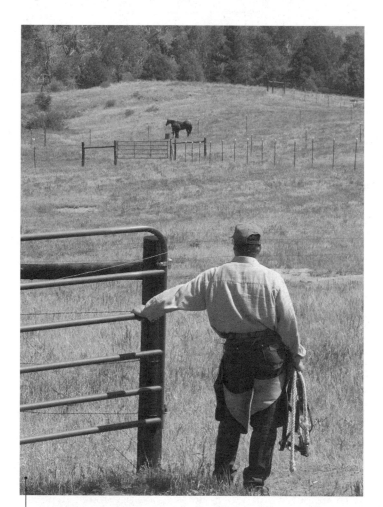

Valuable Time
A farrier's job description does not include hiking across the pasture to gather up your horse. Like your dentist, your doctor, or your veterinarian, your farrier's time is valuable, and many people rely on his services every day. Have your horse ready when the farrier arrives, and he'll have more time to devote to the care of your horse's feet.

Richard says . . .

SKILLS MATTER MOST

A farrier's gender is not important — some fine farriers are men, and others are women. While there's no denying that shoeing horses is hard work, strength takes a back seat to talent, dedication, and skill. We use the pronoun "he" in this book when referring to farriers just as we use "he" when referring to a horse. "He" includes all men and women, stallions, mares, and geldings.

Characteristics of the Ideal Farrier

The best farrier is a true craftsman, one who has a genuine interest in the well-being of horses and pride in his work. He takes the time to polish his skills and looks upon each hoof that he shoes as one that will bear his trademark and demonstrate the quality of his work.

He is a good manager of time and dependable about keeping appointments. A farrier who is routinely late or who cancels appointments causes inconvenience and frustration for horse owners and irregular care for the horses. A farrier must be careful not to pack his day so full that he is in a hurry to keep on schedule, because then he will not do his best work. If the entire week is made up of one frantic hour after another, there is no time to respond to emergencies or replace lost shoes.

He is a good horseman. He understands and is comfortable using standard horse handling methods. Although it is important to stay flexible regarding specific practices at various barns, a good farrier will not consent to work in unsafe conditions or on an untrained horse. A good horseman knows when to say *no*.

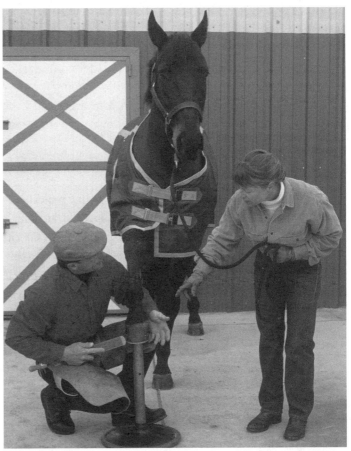

Don't be afraid to ask questions. That's how you learn.

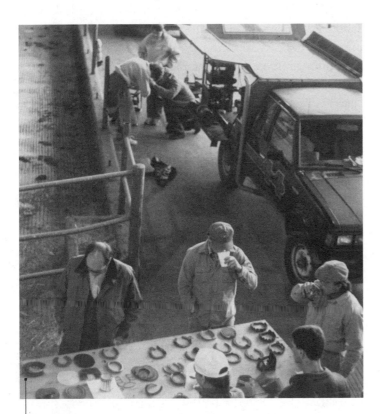

Always Learning
A keen farrier wants to stay abreast of the latest research and developments in hoof-care technology and is able to distinguish solid principles from passing fads. A farrier that does not stay updated is outdated.

Richard says . . .

HOOF CARE ISN'T A DO-IT-YOURSELF JOB

Should you trim and shoe your own horse? You can try, but if you want the best care for your horse, I don't recommend it. There are courses that purport to teach horse owners in a few hours or days how to trim their horse's hooves. But if you want to learn how to trim your horse properly, take a respected farrier course that runs for at least six weeks and that emphasizes anatomy.

It takes a graduate farrier five to seven years of full-time work experience to attain the skills necessary to properly assess, trim, and shoe most horses. And even an experienced farrier will occasionally need advice from other farriers. Either become a professional farrier yourself or secure the services of the best farrier you can afford.

FINDING A FARRIER

The farrier that will best suit you depends on a number of factors. When seeking a horseshoer, consider your level of riding, your activity, your horse's specific shoeing requirements, the pool of farriers available in your area, and your budget. Use a combination of the following methods to identify the most suitable farrier for you.

Solicit Recommendations

Ask five to ten horse people which farriers they would recommend. Try to get a variety of opinions from veterinarians, trainers, other horse owners, and barn managers. Find out which farriers your vet has worked with, how capably each farrier solved problems, and if the farriers worked cooperatively with the horse owners to develop an effective hoof-management program. Ask your veterinarian to name not only the farriers he recommends but also those he does not recommend. Ask several other equine veterinarians in your area for their recommendations as well.

Ask a handful of professional trainers, riding instructors, stable managers, and breeders in your community about their experience with local farriers and about those they currently employ. However, don't value one person's opinion so strongly that you automatically hire or discredit a farrier from a single testimony. Just keep summarizing your findings, paying attention to details such as, "He's really nice, but he's never on time," or "My horses are always ready to step right into the show ring," or "He always gets into a fight with my horse." Ask how long it takes for each farrier to replace lost shoes, if a horse has ever been lame right after shoeing and what the farrier did about it, if the farrier works well with the farm veterinar-ian, and if the farrier gets along well with horses.

If you are a casual trail rider, it would be inappropriate to ask the rider of Grand Prix jumping horses for a farrier recommendation. Instead, find people whose level of management, amount of time spent riding, and riding activities are similar to yours. Ask them the same sorts of questions that you asked the professionals.

Read Advertisements

Check newspapers and bulletin boards, but don't rely solely on printed advertisements. Although some farriers you see advertised might be very qualified, others could be very poorly qualified. No matter what their ads say, they may create long-term problems for you and your horse. Keep in mind that many of the best farriers use only word-of-mouth advertising.

Refer to Farrier Directories

There are many horseshoeing programs throughout the United States. Some courses are part of the curriculum at colleges and universities, while independent horseshoeing schools offer others. The programs range in length from one week to one year or longer. Most programs issue a certificate or diploma upon completion. Some farriers, after attending one of these programs, will list themselves as a "certified farrier" (having completed the certificate program) or a "graduate farrier" (having graduated from a program). However, the qualifications of two farriers who call themselves "certified" could be as different as night and day.

To help rate the skills of U.S. farriers (whether or not they've attended a farrier school), three U.S. organizations offer voluntary testing and certification programs: the American Farrier's Association (AFA), the Brotherhood of Working Farriers Association (BWFA), and the Guild of Professional Farriers (GPF). Applicants to these associations are required to pass written and/or oral exams and demonstrate practical shoeing skills. The testing and grading guidelines vary among these three associations.

Each group maintains a directory of farriers' names, addresses, phone numbers, and levels of certification. By contacting the AFA, the BWFA, or the GPF (see Resource Guide), you can obtain the names of certified farriers in your area. Remember, however, that testing is voluntary, so if you rely solely on membership lists, you may miss finding a very capable farrier who lives just down the road from you but isn't a member of any association.

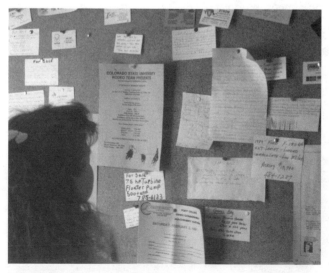

Scan bulletin boards for the names of farriers in your area.

WHY YOU NEED A VETERINARIAN

An equine veterinarian can help you manage your horse's overall health, as well as his leg and hoof soundness. He is also your best contact for advice and treatment related to lameness, wounds, foal hoof management, and nutrition. Whenever a hoof injury involves sensitive tissue — a hot nail, a puncture, an abscess, a bleeding crack, or a coronary band wound, for example — it is important that your veterinarian be involved in the treatment. Although your farrier may perform the actual work (paring an abscess, relieving or resecting a crack, treating a hot nail) it should be done under a veterinarian's supervision. Your veterinarian and farrier should both be involved in prepurchase health evaluations and in helping you formulate a management program for your horse.

FINDING AN EQUINE VETERINARIAN

Locating the skilled equine veterinarian that's right for you and your horse is similar to finding a good farrier. Ask for recommendations from horse owners, farriers, and other professional horse people in your area. Narrow your list to three candidates, and call them to see which ones are accepting new clients.

The American Association of Equine Practitioners (AAEP) has a guide to finding veterinarians on their Web site at www.aaep.org.

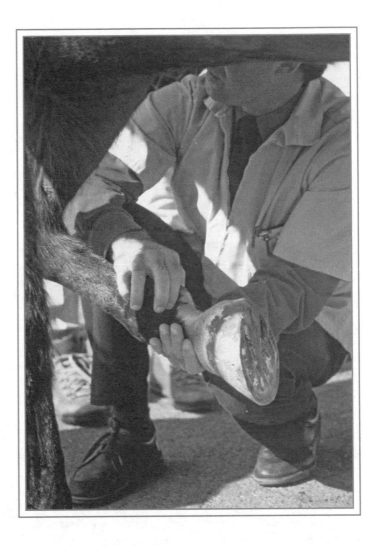

WHOSE JOB?

The job descriptions of farriers, veterinarians, and owners sometimes overlap, and when hooves are involved, confusion and disagreement about who should perform specific procedures can cause friction and make working together difficult. It is usually best if all of the members of your hoof-care team are informed of significant changes and developments regarding your horse's feet.

Example 1: Pulling a shoe. If you or your vet needs to pull a shoe to examine a foot for injury or lameness, you should do so only if you can ensure the hoof will not be damaged in the process and that the hoof can be protected until a farrier arrives to reset the shoe. Otherwise, call your farrier to pull the shoe before you carry out the exam.

Example 2: Hoof injury. Anytime you or your farrier discovers a wound or injury that bleeds or involves sensitive tissue — a cut, a sole abscess, a puncture wound, or an embedded object — consult with your veterinarian for advice and treatment.

Example 3: Lameness. Lameness can have many causes. An unnoticeable puncture, a sore back, and poor shoeing are just some of the conditions that result in lameness. Some farriers know more about hoof anatomy and function than many vets do, and often a proper trim and shoes will set a horse right. However, an equine veterinarian is better trained and equipped to examine the entire horse when diagnosing lameness. Whom you contact first matters little if you've done a good job selecting your team.

-3-

FACILITIES

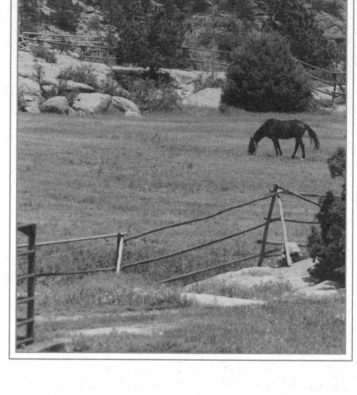

Horse facilities include horse housing, pens, arenas, and outbuildings. The design and condition of your horse facilities can have a big impact on the condition of your horse's feet and hooves. Horses evolved as nomads, traveling freely over abrasive, semiarid grass plains. If you use this native environment as a model for your facilities, your horse will be more comfortable and will perform better, and your farrier and veterinary bills will be minimized.

KEEP THEM DRY

Above all, the areas where your horse lives — pastures, pens, and stalls — should have well-drained footing.

Standing for long periods in water or wet footing is one of the top causes of hoof problems. Excess moisture softens the tough outer hoof wall, allowing it to deform into flares and to develop cracks more easily. A waterlogged hoof can separate into layers, and dirt, gravel, and bacteria can invade the hoof, breaking it down even further. A sole that is softened by too much moisture will bruise more easily than a hard, dry sole; this can lead to abscesses and lameness. Hoof diseases like thrush and white line disease thrive in the dark, damp recesses of dirty hooves.

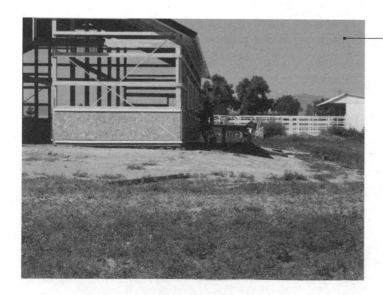

Higher Is Drier

Before building, properly prepare the site for your barn so that the soil and other materials beneath the floor percolate well. Ideally, the finished level of the barn site should be 8 to 12 inches (20.3–30.5 cm) above ground level. At that height, snowmelt and rain runoff drain away from the barn. If the existing soil is well drained, the site can be prepared by the addition of 6 inches (15.2 cm) of crushed rock covered by soil.

Your local extension agent or planning department can help you test the percolation rate of your soil (how fast water drains through it), help you design the excavation, and suggest a fill that will be suitable for your soil.

STALL FLOORING

Flooring and bedding make up the footing of your horse's stall. Flooring should be comfortable for the horse, whether he's standing or lying down. The best flooring minimizes stress on a horse's feet and legs. It should have sufficient traction, especially when wet, so a person or a horse won't slip and be injured. It should provide a surface that is easy to clean and keep dry so the hooves are not subjected to excess moisture. No matter what flooring you choose, proper preparation and careful installation of the stall base are critical. There are basically two types of stall floorings: draining and nondraining.

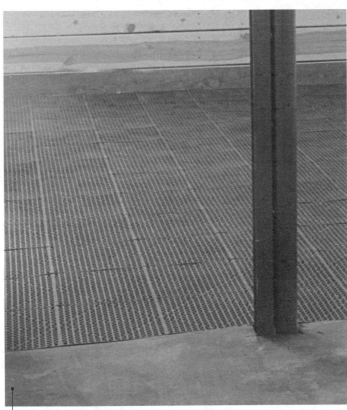

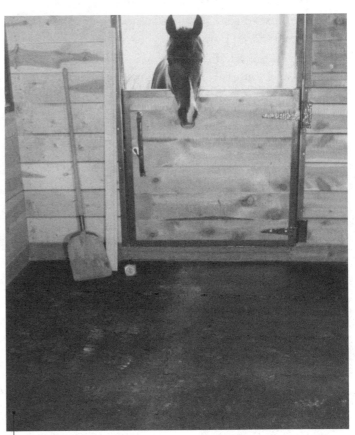

Draining Flooring

Draining flooring consists of porous tiles or mats that allow urine to pass through to the ground below. This type of flooring reduces bedding costs because only the bedding immediately around the urine stream becomes wet and is discarded. With draining flooring, the subfloor soil beneath the stall must drain very well to a depth of several feet. Otherwise, the accumulation of urine underneath the flooring can be a source of foul odors and ammonia, an unhealthy gas, and will require excavation and replacement of the saturated soil.

Solid Flooring

A nondraining solid flooring is made of a nonpermeable material that keeps moisture on top of it. With this type of flooring, the urine and moisture are soaked up by bedding and removed regularly. Consequently, more bedding is used. For a barn on poorly drained soils, consider nondraining flooring and plan to clean stalls more often. Remove wet bedding as soon as possible to help your horse's hooves stay dry.

MORE STALLS THAN HORSES

One thing that will make stall flooring longer lasting and healthier for your horses is to have more stalls in your barn than you do horses. This enables you to rotate horses among the stalls so the flooring can dry out thoroughly between uses.

When deciding on stall flooring, keep in mind initial cost and labor versus long-term maintenance and replacement cost. Using top quality materials and careful installation practices may seem extravagant at the outset, but they can end up saving you time and money, especially if your stalls are going to see a lot of use.

NATURAL MATERIALS
(dirt, clay, sand, gravel, road base)

Pros: Inexpensive; provide some cushion; have good traction without being overly abrasive

Cons: Readily softened by urine and spilled water; holes and humps form where horses paw or habitually stand and turn; slow to dry, hold odors, difficult to clean; can be dusty; small gravel can become imbedded in moisture-softened hooves, causing abscesses; a horse eating off the stall floor can ingest sand or dirt, which can lead to the life-threatening condition known as sand colic

CONCRETE, ASPHALT

Pros: Long-lasting; easy to maintain

Cons: Abrasive to hooves; fatiguing for a horse to stand on; requires very deep bedding to be comfortable or safe for a horse to lie on

WOOD

Pros: Rustic ambience; relatively inexpensive

Cons: Difficult to clean and sanitize because the surface is porous and usually uneven; holds unpleasant odors; slippery when wet

DRAINING FLOORING
(porous tiles and mats)

Pros: Long-lasting; easy to clean; minimizes bedding use; some provide good cushion

Cons: Accumulation of urine under the flooring can lead to odor problems; open-grid design of some is filled with a layer of sand or dirt, which exposes a horse to risk of colic from ingestion

SOLID RUBBER MATS

Pros: Provide a firm, level surface with cushion; low maintenance; long-lasting; when used with absorbent bedding, allow moisture from urine to be removed with bedding at each stall cleaning

Cons: Some are heavy to handle when installing; can buckle or separate at the joints if not installed properly; some can be slippery when wet

WATERPROOF STALL MATTRESS

Pros: Provides cushion for standing and lying; is impermeable to moisture, so the subfloor stays dry; uses less bedding than rubber mats because it is only needed for absorption, not for cushion

Cons: Stall-doorway thresholds may need to be modified for proper installation of mattress

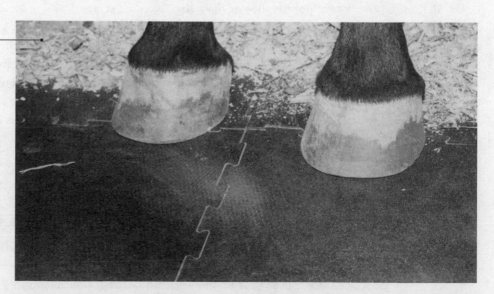

Interlocking Rubber Mats
Interlocking solid rubber mats can make an excellent stall floor. When installed over a properly prepared base, the mats act like a one-piece floor with no buckling or separating. Little or no urine is able to seep through the joints and under the flooring.

TYPES OF BEDDING

- **Sand** makes comfortable bedding for a horse to stand and lie on. It is often used in animal hospitals for horses that have laminitis because it enables a horse to stand with his painful feet at the angle that is most comfortable and least damaging.

  A big drawback to sand bedding is that it increases the risk of sand colic. Colic is the leading cause of death in horses. Sometimes a horse intentionally eats sand because his diet is deficient in minerals. A horse in a sand stall will ingest a significant amount of sand while eating hay off the floor.

- **Straw** is available almost everywhere and is perhaps the most traditional horse bedding. It makes an inviting nest for a horse to lie in, and when composted it decomposes quickly.

  On the downside, straw doesn't absorb odors or moisture as well as other types of bedding and it can be slippery underfoot. When wet, straw packs into the horse's feet and is tracked onto the barn aisle. Good bedding is often thrown out with the bad when a stall is cleaned because it's difficult to separate clean straw from manure and wet straw.

  Many horses like to eat oat straw used for bedding, which can adversely affect their health and weight. Oat straw also tends to become slimy and slippery when wet. Wheat straw, because of its high glaze, does not become as slimy as oat straw, but it is less absorbent. Because it's less palatable, it's a better choice for a horse that overeats. Barley straw should be avoided because of the sharp, barbed awns that can become lodged in a horse's gums.

- **Wood products such as sawdust, chips, and shavings** are available in bulk in timber country and packaged almost everywhere. Softwood products tend to be more absorbent than hardwood. The thinner and smaller the shavings, the softer and more absorbent the bedding will be — and the more it will end up in the horse's coat, mane, and tail. Fine sawdust can fill the air with dust and can ball up in the horse's feet when wet.

- **Hardwood products** are not desirable for bedding because of their poor absorbency and because they are more likely to cause allergic reactions in horses. Avoid black walnut in particular because it is toxic to horses. Many horses that have contacted black walnut shavings quickly contracted laminitis and died.

- **Shredded paper** from newspapers and phone books (not magazines, computer paper, or colored pages) makes very absorbent bedding, and it decomposes as quickly as straw when composted. The ink used by U.S. newspapers is soy-based, so it likely won't harm horses that eat it, but it can stain the coats of light-colored horses. When dry, paper bedding is very flammable, and when wet it compacts into dense layers that can make cleaning a stall difficult.

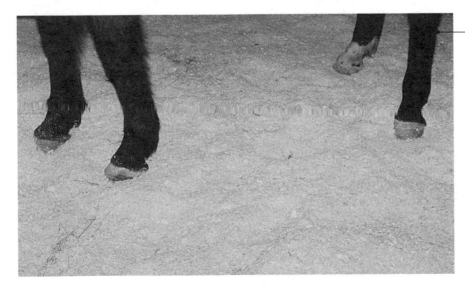

Clean, Dry Bedding for Healthy Hooves
Bedding provides cushion for a horse's feet and legs; gives him a soft, dry place to lie down; and absorbs moisture, especially urine, so it can be removed from the stall. Even the best bedding can add to hoof problems if it is wet and not removed frequently.

With bulk bedding like sawdust that hasn't been cleaned and packaged, be on the lookout for foreign objects such as wire, nails, and splinters that could get lodged in a horse's feet or injure him when he lies down to rest.

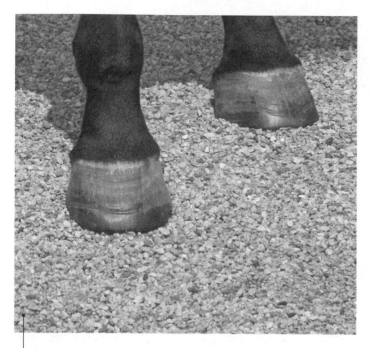

Well-Drained Pen

In order for a pen to provide good footing in all types of weather, it should be located on solid ground that slopes at least ¼ inch per foot (0.64 cm per 0.3 m) away from the pen. That way rain and snowmelt will drain out of and away from the pen. The top layer of footing should be a material such as small gravel that will minimize mud.

Richard says . . .

DRYING OUT IS WORTH THE EFFORT

I've seen many hoof problems over the years that were caused by horses' feet being too wet. Although management situations sometimes made it difficult to move a horse from wet footing to dry ground, doing so always improved the condition of the hooves. That's why I recommend you do what you can to keep the feet dry.

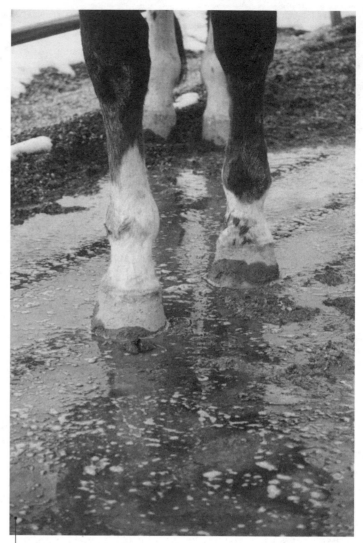

Wet Pens Are Bad for Hooves

A dirt pen that has little or no slope quickly develops a depression in the center and a ridge around the perimeter from the horse's movements. During wet weather, such a pen then turns into a muddy wallow that is very damaging to hooves. To maintain proper drainage, periodically use a rake or shovel to pull the ridge of material that builds up along the perimeter of the pen back into the center and use it to fill low spots.

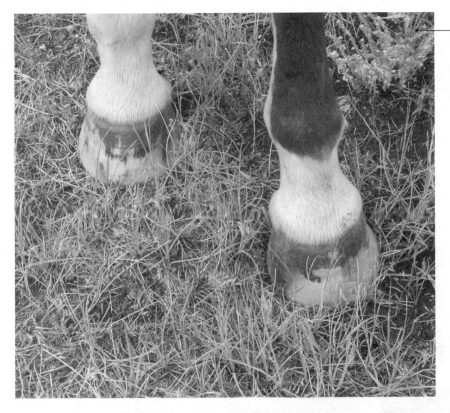

Dry Pasture Is Ideal

A dry pasture is a great place for a horse to exercise, graze, roll, and just be a horse. The natural footing will help condition bare hooves, and the grass will buff the hoof walls of bare or shod feet to a healthy gloss.

Keep Horses Off Wet Pasture

When a pasture gets wet from precipitation or irrigation, or if it is a seasonal wetland, it is best if the horse is brought into a well-drained pen until the pasture dries out. This will prevent unnecessary damage to the pasture and help maintain the health of the horse's hooves.

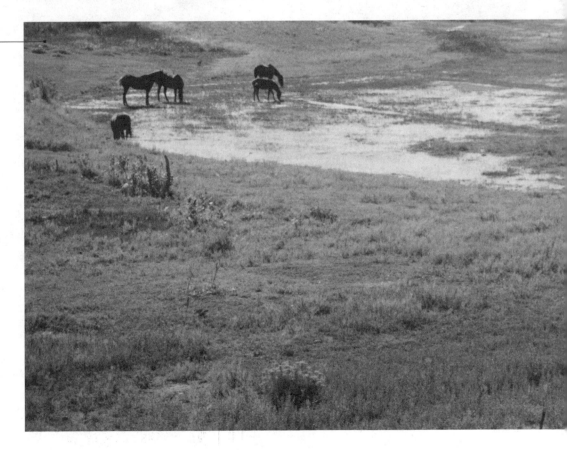

WORK AREAS

To enable your farrier to do his very best work, provide a proper shoeing area that is well lit and uncluttered. Its smooth, level surface can be concrete, rubber, wood, or asphalt. Since many farriers require electricity for tools and lights, the shoeing area should be within easy reach of a 110-volt electrical outlet.

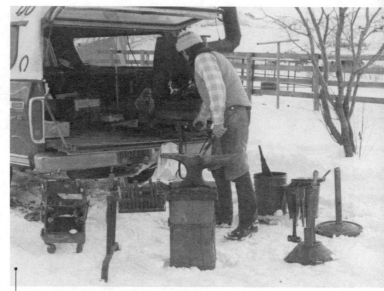

No Snow Shoeing

Your farrier should not be expected to shoe on a gravel driveway, out in the middle of a pasture, in a muddy or rocky paddock, or in snow. Shoeing on rough, uneven ground makes it very difficult for him to see if the hooves are balanced, and it often makes it difficult for the horse to stand comfortably or squarely. A freshly trimmed unprotected hoof set down on gravel can be damaged in a split second.

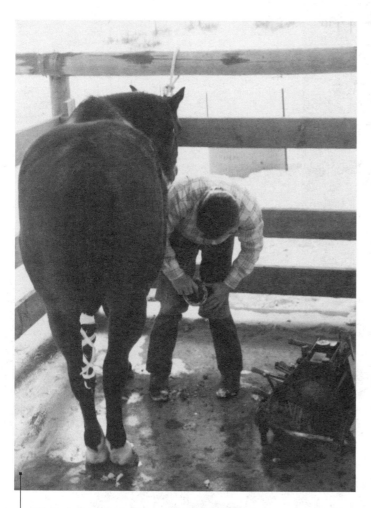

Maintain an Outdoor Shoeing Area

Your farrier may have personal opinions about the type of floor he prefers or whether he likes to work in a small enclosure or a large open area. Your facility may not be his ideal, but the least you can do is provide a dry surface out of the weather. Some farriers prefer to work in a shaded outdoor area to take advantage of cooling breezes and fresh air.

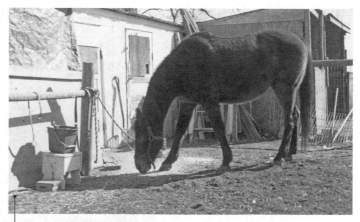

Clutter Spells Danger

Working on a horse in a cluttered area like this is dangerous for both the horse and the farrier. In addition, the horse is tied too low and too long. If he moved suddenly, he could knock something over that could injure him or frighten him into pulling back.

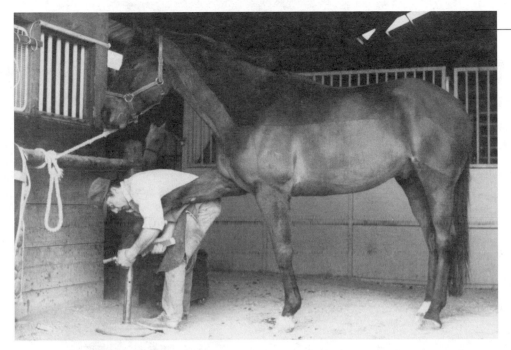

Tie Rail Too Low
Some farriers prefer to work on the horse while he's tied at a hitch rail or in cross-ties. The tie area should be strong and safe. When tied to a hitch rail, the horse should be tied at or above the level of the withers with 2 to 3 feet (0.6–0.9 m) of rope between the halter and the post. The short rope and low rail shown here prevent the horse from attaining a comfortable head position and make it difficult and dangerous for the farrier to bring the horse's front legs forward for work.

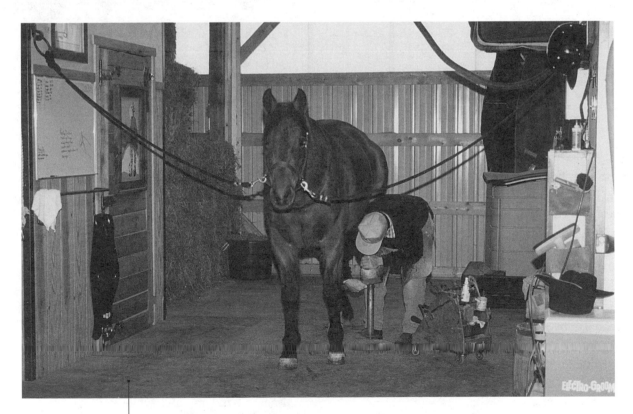

Cross-Ties Provide Ample Room to Work
The height of cross-ties will vary according to the width of the alley spanned. Very wide alleys require long cross-ties mounted high; cross-ties in narrow alleys are shorter and can be mounted so the ties are at about the horse's eye level.

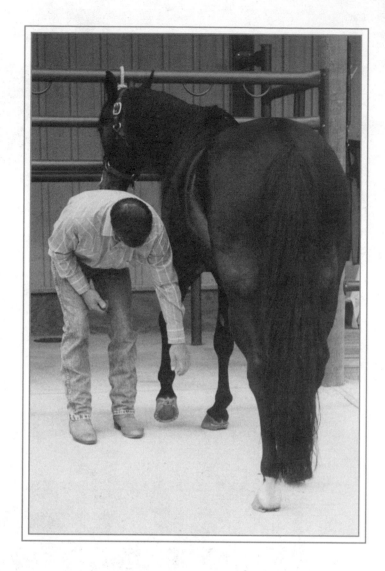

-4-
TRAINING

If you train your horses to be cooperative and relaxed for hoof and leg handling, your farrier and vet will be able to do their best work and will look forward to coming back to your barn. It is not your farrier's or your vet's job to train your horse. And it is unfair to expect them to risk injury or take extra time to handle an untrained horse. If you raise horses, begin hoof handling when they are very young — that early training will last a lifetime. If you purchase a horse that has bad manners, take the time to give him progressive lessons or get professional assistance. See the Resource Guide for recommended training publications.

Before hiring a farrier or vet, be certain your horse has learned all of these lessons:

- Giving to pressure on the poll from your fingers or a halter and lowering the head
- Giving to pressure on the poll and throat latch from a halter and moving forward

- Standing tied without pulling back
- Standing still while tied, unless asked to move
- Standing tied without pawing
- Picking up all four feet cooperatively while haltered and held in hand and also while tied
- Standing in balance for two minutes when any leg is held, without fidgeting, nibbling, moving, leaning, or trying to pull his leg away
- Moving sideways to the left and right on cue, one step at a time, while haltered and held in hand and also while tied
- Backing up and stepping forward on cue, one step at a time, in hand and also while tied
- Allowing all four legs to be brought backward
- Allowing all four legs to be brought forward on a hoof stand (see page 42) or your knee for at least a minute

EARLY HOOF-HANDLING LESSONS

On the first day of the foal's life, begin to accustom him to being caught and having his body and legs handled. When the foal is a week old, you should be able to pick up a leg and hold it while a competent handler holds the foal with a halter alongside the stall wall or a sturdy fence. (It is best to have the mare nearby to give the foal confidence.)

At first just pick up the foal's legs briefly, but increase the amount of time to at least 30 seconds per leg. You should be able to achieve this goal within a week with daily practice. Eventually, you should be able to hold a leg up for two to three minutes. This will condition the foal to stand still long enough for the farrier to trim his hooves.

When you can hold a leg without the foal struggling, gently bend the hoof from side to side and from front to back. This accustoms the foal to the movements farriers make when trimming.

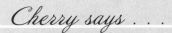

Cherry says . . .

EARLY TRAINING IS KEY

It's important to start foal training early but even more important to review the lessons regularly, throughout a horse's life.

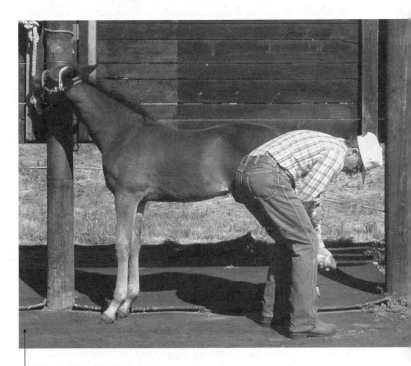

Start 'Em Young
Many foals require corrective rasping to balance their hooves at two months of age or earlier. To prepare the foal for the farrier's first visit, hold a regular series of hoof-handling lessons.

Training Pays Off for Life
Here's the same horse, years later, standing comfortably for the farrier. A properly trained foal will retain his farrier-friendly manners through-out his life. For safety's sake, regularly review leg-handling lessons with all horses to rein-force their good manners and ease the farrier's work.

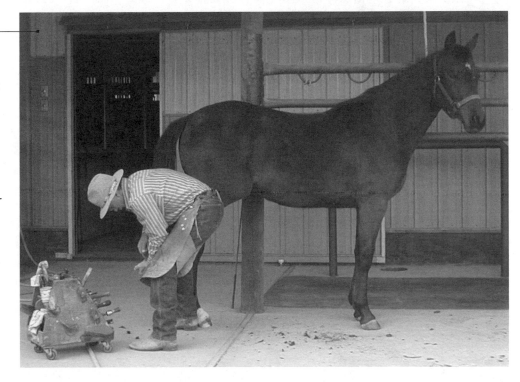

TRAINING GUIDELINES FOR HOOF HANDLING

To be sure that a horse of any age is comfortable having his legs handled and that the lessons proceed safely, follow the guidelines below.

Work in close to the horse's body. This helps restrain the horse, gives the horse an added measure of confidence, and is safer for the handler.

Use generous shoulder-to-shoulder or shoulder-to-hip body contact with the horse to assure him that your control is not tenuous. Do not, however, allow or encourage your horse to lean on you. Although it may not be difficult to support part of the body weight of a 100-pound foal, it won't be long before that foal is a 1,200-pound animal. If a horse starts to lean, let his weight suddenly fall while still holding the foot. He'll quickly learn to support his weight on three legs.

Minimize the amount of sideways pull you exert on the horse's leg. Try to lift the leg in the plane in which it normally moves; that is, underneath the horse's body. With a tiny foal, this may require you to crouch down to the foal's level.

Never let your horse decide when it is time to put his foot down. You choose the moment. It should be when the horse is standing quietly, not struggling. Then place the hoof decisively on the ground (don't let it just drop).

If a horse does try to pull his leg away from you, you will have a better chance of hanging on if you tip the toe up so the fetlock and pastern are hyperflexed. This tends to block nerve transmissions and reflexes.

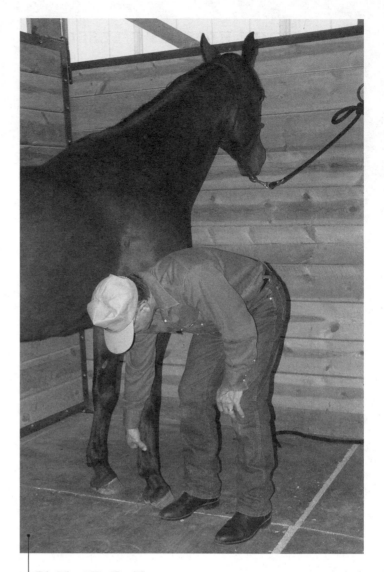

Picking Up the Feet

When you are picking up a right leg, push the horse's weight over to the horse's left shoulder or hip with your shoulder or elbow. Don't try to pick up a hoof by force. Rather, take advantage of the horse's inborn withdrawal reflex.

When a branch or a buzzing fly touches a wild horse's leg, the horse's automatic reaction is to pick up his leg, often very quickly and high. Your domestic horse will still exhibit this reflex, especially if you touch the leg in a strategic area. But because you will also want to be able to groom, bandage, and clip your horse's legs without his picking them up, you can teach him to differentiate between your command (such as *foot*) to pick up a foot and the one that tells him to keep his feet on the ground (such as *stand on it*).

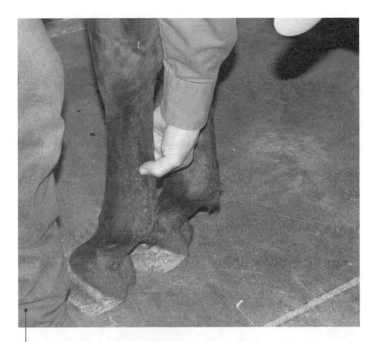

Use the Tendon Reflex

To teach a horse to pick up his foot, give the voice command, *foot*, while at the same time pinching the tendon area above the fetlock. This will cause most horses to reflexively pick up the foot.

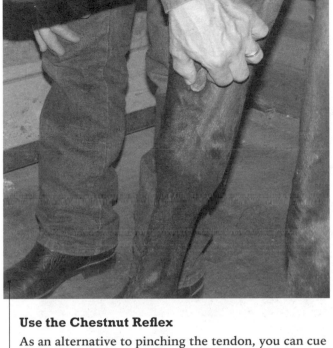

Use the Chestnut Reflex

As an alternative to pinching the tendon, you can cue the horse to pick up his front foot by squeezing the chestnut, the horny growth on the inside of the leg above the knee on a front leg.

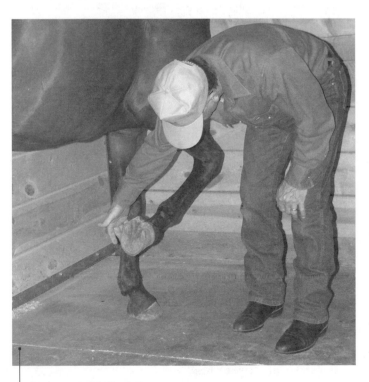

Just a Light Touch

Within a short time your horse will respond to a very light touch or the voice command alone.

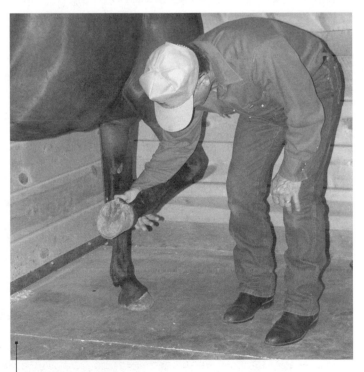

Catch and Hold the Hoof

As your horse lifts his foot you should be ready to catch and hold it. Otherwise, he'll put it right back down as part of the reflex cycle.

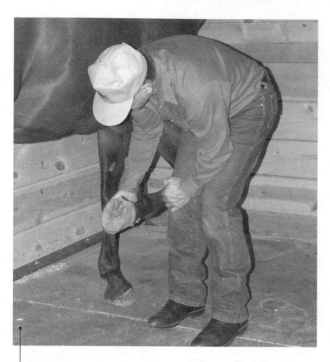

Owner Position for Front Leg Held Back

For everyday cleaning and inspection, hold the hoof in one hand and the cleaning tools in the other hand. Once you have grasped the hoof, hold it in a natural position without pulling the leg outward or overflexing the joints. If the process is made comfortable for a horse, especially a foal, he will be less likely to struggle.

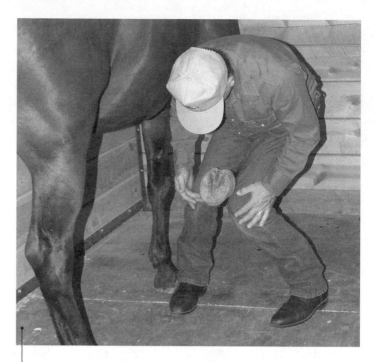

Farrier Position for Front Leg Held Back

When working on a front foot, the farrier will need to hold the foot between his knees in order to have both hands free to handle his tools. When practicing this position with your horse, you may have to crouch and adjust your stance in order to keep the leg under his body and not pulled out to the side. This likely will be more difficult for you than it is for your horse.

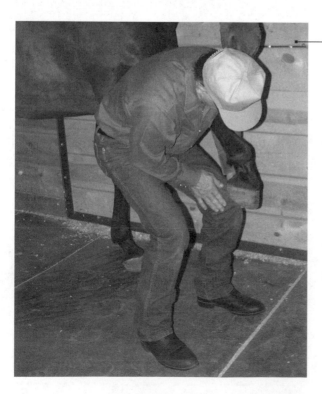

Forward Farrier Position for Front Leg Held Forward

Once your horse is comfortable having his front feet held back in the normal trimming position, bring the leg forward and rest it on your knee or on a hoof stand. You can bring the foot forward from the ground or you can bring the foot back first and then bring it forward — whichever action is most comfortable. When using a hoof stand (see page 42), always maintain contact with the foot to prevent it from slipping off or tipping the stand over. You might want to have a helper hold the horse to keep him from nuzzling and slobbering on your head.

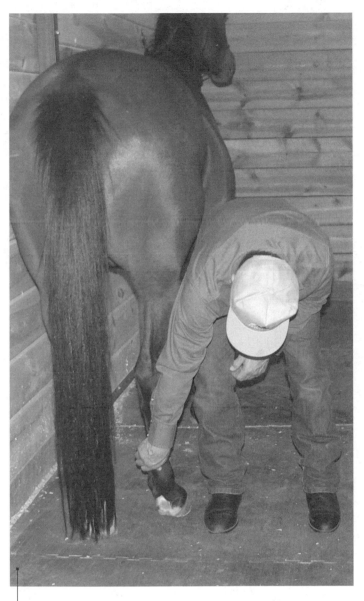

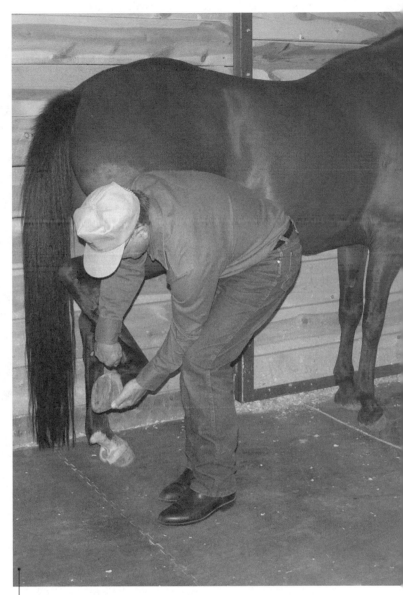

Position for Lifting Hind Feet

When signaling your horse to lift his hind feet, it's usually more convenient and effective to squeeze the tendon than it is to squeeze the chestnut. Stand in close to the horse so he can feel your shoulder on his body. This is the safest position for you if a horse kicks because the hind leg usually swings outward, the way a cow kicks. Get the horse used to standing calmly for a few minutes, as you stand close against his side and flank. Then progress to picking up the foot.

Practice Catching the Hind Foot

Catch the hind foot low when it comes off the ground. It might be easier to maintain control if you hold the foot with both hands at first. If your horse initially makes big leg movements, practice, practice, practice with patience until he calmly lifts his foot.

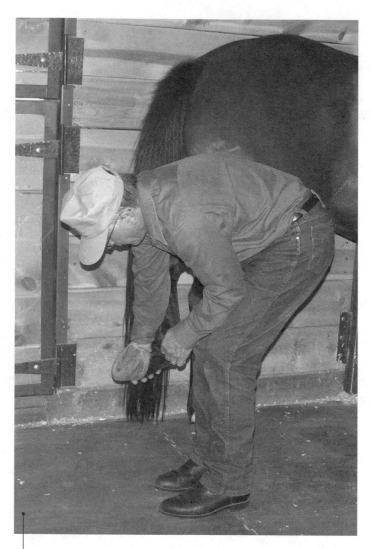

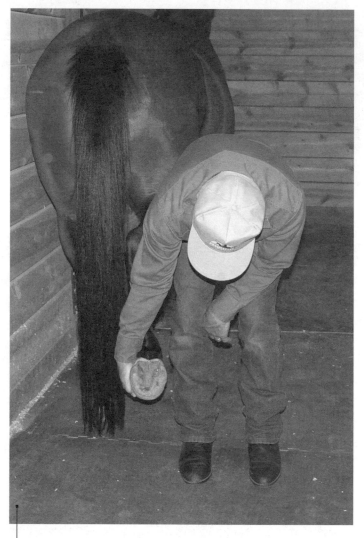

Owner Position for Hind Leg Held Back
For routine hoof cleaning, hold the hoof in one hand, leaving your other hand free to hold the pick.

Hold Hind Hoof Low for Horse's Comfort
As with the front hooves, try to keep the leg in line with its natural plane of movement. Foals, short horses, and arthritic horses usually are most comfortable when the hind leg is held low.

Richard says . . .

HOOF-HANDLING AWARENESS

When handling a horse's feet, make note of what the horse's reactions and movements are telling you. Is he comfortable and relaxed? Frightened and tense? In pain or imbalanced?

As I often hear Cherry say, "The horse will tell you what you need to work on." It's up to you to think like a horse and help your horse learn to be comfortable with hoof handling.

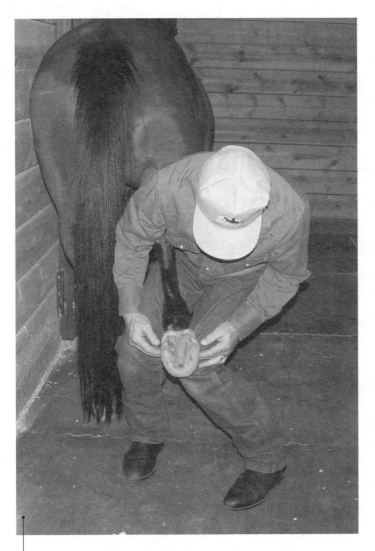

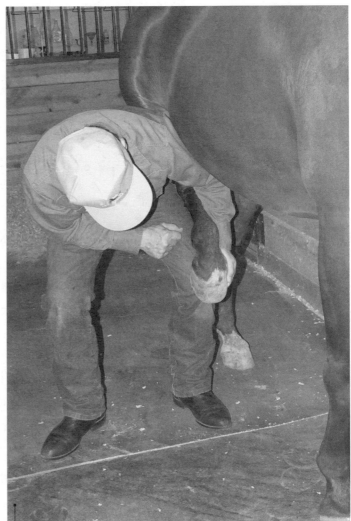

Farrier Position for Hind Leg Held Back

The farrier will need to rest the horse's hoof on his leg or lap in order to have both hands free to use his tools. From the horse owner position, gradually bring your horse's leg up and get him used to resting it on your leg. You may have to crouch to make some horses comfortable with this position. Raising the leg too high just to accommodate the height of your lap may cause the horse discomfort in his joints, especially the stifle. A horse often struggles when his legs are held because his joints are stressed by improper leg lifting.

Farrier Position for Hind Leg Held Forward

The horse also needs to be comfortable bringing his hind leg forward and resting the hoof on your knee or a hoof stand. Be sure the horse isn't a kicker before trying to lift the hoof forward from the ground; you will be facing forward in a vulnerable position. As with the front legs, always maintain contact with the hoof when it is resting on a hoof stand.

-5-

MANAGEMENT

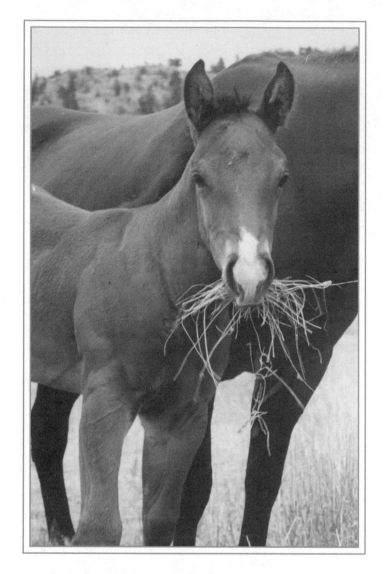

Your overall management program can improve your horse's hoof quality and health. Start by providing your horse with a balanced, natural diet. House your horse in dry, sanitary facilities. Maintain the facilities so they are safe and comfortable. Provide your horse with some type of daily exercise. Make time each day to attend to his grooming including a hoof inspection. Keep your horse on a regular farrier schedule.

A BALANCED DIET

Feeding a balanced ration of grass pasture (if available), hay and grain, and supplements (if needed) is essential for the development and maintenance of healthy hooves.

- Learn the difference between poor- and good-quality hay, and buy the best you can afford.
- Test hay for nutrient content, and add supplements as needed.

- Measure hay and grain by weight, not volume.
- Feed little or no grain.
- Gradually get a horse used to pasture using short, limited turnout periods, and closely monitor his weight and comfort when he's on pasture.
- Maintain your horse at a healthy weight to prevent excess stress on his hooves.
- Do not feed a horse immediately after hard work, and do not work a horse until one hour after a full feeding.
- Provide free-choice trace-mineralized salt, loose or in block form.

After formulating the hay and grain portions of your horse's ration, choose a supplement that provides missing nutrients. A balanced formula is usually better than adding separate nutrients. Frequently, hooves benefit from a formula containing vitamins A and D, lysine, biotin, calcium, selenium, and zinc. With this formula, your horse's hair coat also may improve, as it is composed of proteins similar to those found in the hooves.

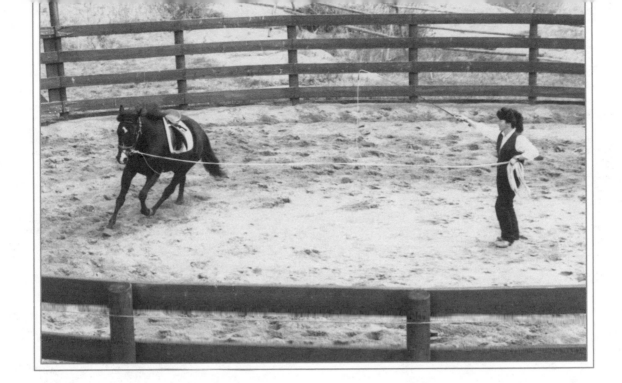

EXERCISE FOR STRONG HOOVES

Exercise will benefit overall health and is essential for the proper development of bones and dense, tough hooves. Horses of all ages need exercise every day. Exercise can improve the quality and strength of bones, tendons, ligaments, and hooves and speed healing of damaged tissue. Regular, moderate stress creates dense, stress-resistant bones and hooves. Exercise also conditions and stretches muscles and tendons, lessening the chance of injury and lameness. If your horse stands inactive for long periods of time, the blood may not deliver sufficient moisture to the hooves, and they may contract.

It is important that the footing in the exercise area is not too deep. Hyperextension of the fetlock in deep sand, for example, can do permanent damage to tendons. Rough and rocky footing can encourage the development of dense, tough hooves but can also cause hoof damage, especially if the horse's hooves are soft and weak when he is first turned out on that sort of terrain.

Riding is an ideal way to provide daily exercise for a horse (and rider!), as it can be controlled yet varied. Turn-out on pasture is the least labor intensive and most natural way of providing exercise. However, many horses choose not to exercise when left to their own devices. They prefer to spend most of their time eating when turned out onto pasture, or simply turn into "gate potatoes," waiting to be brought back in. That's why it is important to design a varied exercise program and ensure your horses get a daily workout. On days when you can't ride or drive them, there are other options.

Alternatives to Riding

If your horse doesn't exercise on his own, there are other ways to keep his heart, bones, and hooves healthy:

Ponying, leading one horse while riding another, is a good way to exercise two horses and one rider at the same time. This can be done in an arena or in open spaces on varied terrain.

Longeing is an option best suited for horses over two years of age. Because of repeated, uneven loading of the limbs associated with circle work, younger horses may suffer sprains and strains from excessive longeing, especially in small circles. For any age horse, it is ideal if the longe circle is 66 feet (20 m) in diameter.

Electric horse walkers are useful for warm-ups and occasional exercise sessions but should not be viewed as the mainstay of a horse's exercise program. Thirty minutes of walking once or twice a week is a good alternative if on those days the horse would otherwise have to stand in a stall. Depending entirely on a walker for exercise, however, can be boring for the horse and encourage undesirable habits such as a stiff carriage, resistance, and laziness.

Treadmills can be used for an occasional workout if the horse is gradually conditioned to the work and carefully monitored for signs of stress. A continuous climb at the 5- to 7-degree slope characteristic of most treadmills can be extremely fatiguing. A workout using a treadmill is accomplished in about half the time required for most other forms of exercise. Note that a treadmill workout could seriously strain the tendons of a horse with long toes and low heels.

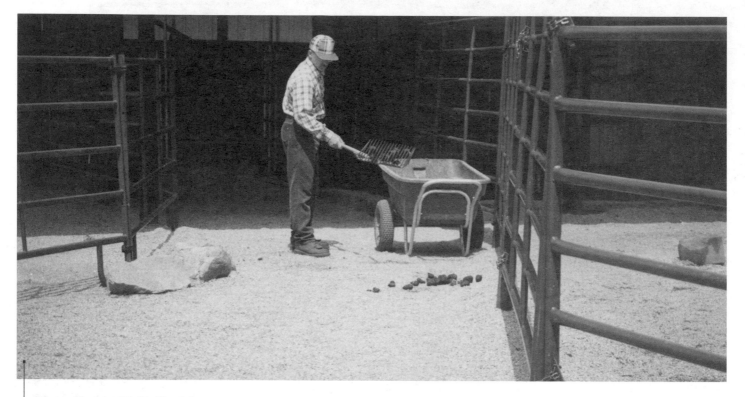

Clean Pens and Stalls Often

Diligent sanitation practices are essential for hoof health. A 1,000-pound horse produces approximately 50 pounds of manure and 6 gallons of urine per day. As these waste products break down, they release ammonia, which is harmful not only to hooves but also to eyes, skin, and the respiratory system. Also, bedding wet with dung and urine provides a perfect environment for the proliferation of bacteria and fungi that can break down the hoof wall, frog, and sole. To prevent ammonia formation and to keep your horse from standing in unhealthy footing, the manure and wet bedding should be collected several times a day — once a day at the very least. Disposal options include having it hauled away, spreading it immediately on a pasture or arena, or storing it for later spreading.

Keep the Stall Floor Dry

If your horse is kept in a stall, clean the stall often and if possible leave the floor uncovered to air dry. If the stall is to be used again immediately, sprinkle an odor-neutralizing and drying product over the wet areas. Products made from zeolites are safe and effective. Avoid hydrated lime (barn lime); although it traditionally has been used to dry stalls, it is strongly alkaline and can be harmful to people and horses.

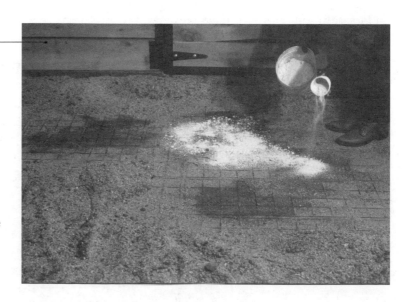

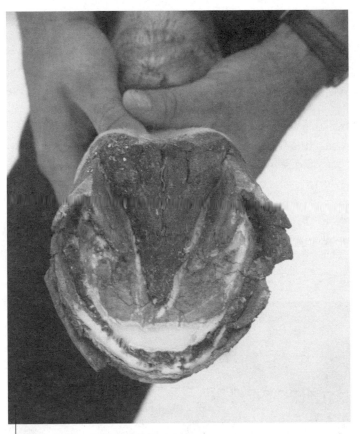

Hoof Deteriorated by Too Much Moisture

Hooves softened by wet bedding, water, mud, frequent baths, or excessive hoof dressing are weak. In this state they often spread out at the bottom and separate into layers.

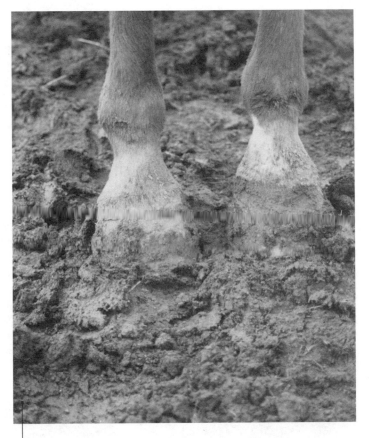

Avoid Mud

Your horse's hooves can be severely damaged if he stands in mud for long periods. Wet mud can soften a hoof excessively, and when mud dries on a hoof, it can draw moisture from the hoof wall and cause cracks. (See page 103.)

Dry Footing Is Best for Hooves

Healthy hooves can usually tolerate brief exposure to water, such as crossing through a creek. But regular or prolonged exposure to moisture can make the hooves very weak and prone to problems. When a horse is kept on dry footing, the hooves have a better chance of remaining hard, tough, and strong.

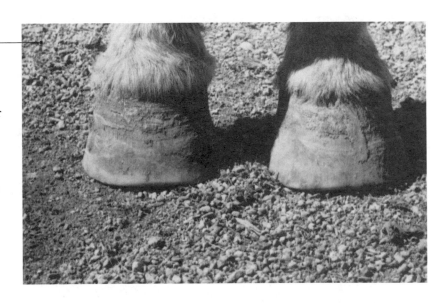

DAILY HOOF CHECK

Establishing a daily routine of closely examining your horse will help you spot health problems quickly and deal with them before they become more serious. Give your horse a visual once-over each day at a regularly scheduled time, if possible, such as during feeding. Your check should include noting your horse's overall stance and attitude, the condition of his legs, how he moves, and clues in his living area such as paw holes or a lost shoe. If you notice something unusual about a leg or hoof, halter your horse and bring him to an area where you can pick out his hooves and give him a close exam.

In order to spot problems, first you need a good sense of what constitutes normal for hooves in general. Each horse has his own normal. Make note of the individual characteristics of each of your own horse's hooves. To establish a baseline for comparison in relation to texture, temperature, and sensitivity of your horse's legs and hooves, be sure to carry out a preliminary examination when your horse is sound. Take note of your horse's bare hooves, or shoes if he's shod, right after the farrier finishes so you'll be able to tell if anything changes.

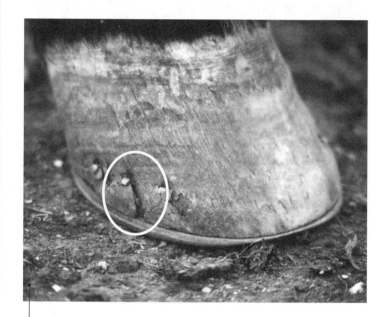

Check the Coronary Band Closely

Look for signs of injury on the coronary band **(A)**, bulbs, and lower leg. Sometimes hair will hide cuts or embedded objects in these areas. This horse has suffered previous coronary-band injuries, as evidenced by two horizontal cracks **(B)** that have grown down with the hoof.

Keep an Eye on Cracks

Wipe any dirt, mud, or manure off the hoof wall and see if any cracks are forming, especially near the nail clinches. If there are existing cracks, check to see if they are changing in size or are growing out normally. Cracks caused by low nails or thick nails, as shown here, can increase in size and lead to lost shoes.

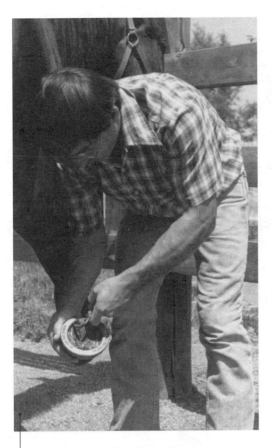

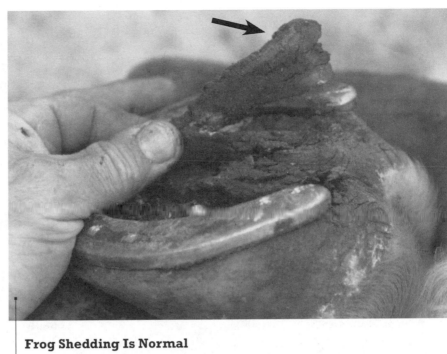

Frog Shedding Is Normal

It is not uncommon for a horse to shed large portions of his frog when it becomes too long or overgrown. This is especially true in damp environments, where the frog is not worn away naturally. Loose flaps of frog are insensitive tissue that can be removed with scissors or a sharp knife.

Clean Each Hoof Carefully

Pick out each hoof. If your horse shows sensitivity in the clefts on either side or in the center of the frog when you clean his feet, it could be a sign of injury or thrush.

Check for Foreign Objects

Look for foreign objects lodged in the sole, frog, or heel bulbs. If a stick or piece of wire seems loose and not embedded, pull it out. If the wound bleeds or if you think the object goes into sensitive tissue, it is often better to leave the object in place and call your veterinarian. That way, when the vet removes the object, he'll be better able to tell if the whole thing came out or if a portion remained in the hoof. He will also be able to immediately treat the open hole left by the removed object.

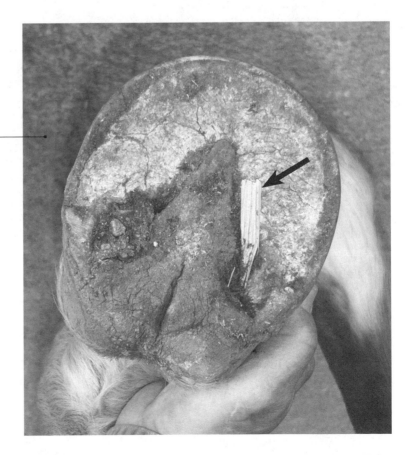

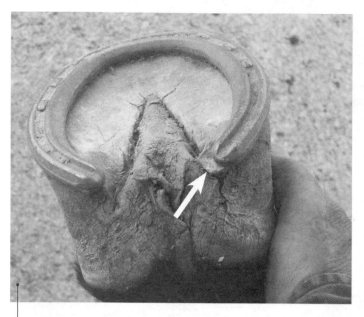

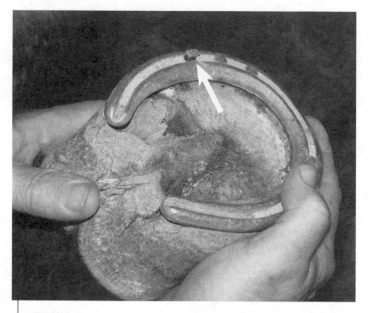

Lodged Stone

Make sure there are no stones or other objects wedged under the heels of the shoe. A lodged stone can bruise the foot and cause an abscess and lameness.

Loose Nail Head

Look closely at the heads of the nails to make sure they are all setting tight in the crease of the shoe. If a nail head appears loose, like this heel nail, either it is time for a reset or the horse may have stepped on the shoe and loosened the nail. Consult your farrier.

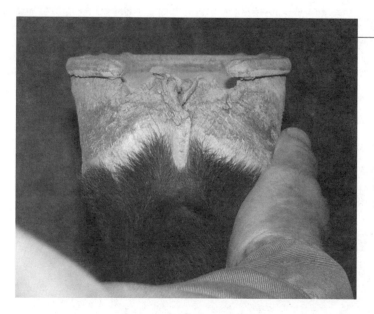

Eyeball the Shoe for Levelness

Sight down the ground surface of the shoe to make sure it is still level. This shoe is level and tight, but sometimes a horse will step on the heel of the shoe and bend it. (See photo on page 98.) This puts uneven stress on the hoof and leg. Even if a bent shoe is still secure on the hoof, contact your farrier. He will remove the shoe, straighten it, and then reset it.

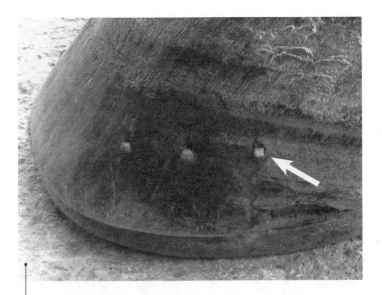

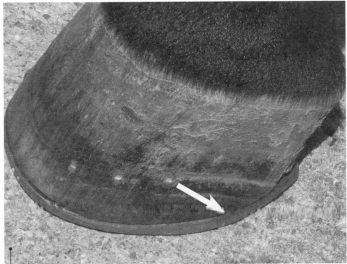

Loose Clinch

Look closely at the clinches to see if they have changed since the horse was shod. If the clinches are no longer flat against the hoof or look as if they are moving up and down in the nail holes, the shoe could be coming loose. It's not uncommon for a horse to catch the heel of the shoe on something and slightly loosen the heel clinch, as in this photo. Look closely and you can see that the clinch no longer blends into the hoof like the other two clinches. In this case, it would be best to check the clinches daily and call the farrier if they become looser. (See page 85 for more about clinches.)

Check Expansion Room

Check how much room for expansion is left on the shoe at the heels. When the hoof has grown out to the edge of the shoe, as the hoof in this photo has, it is usually within a week or two of reset time.

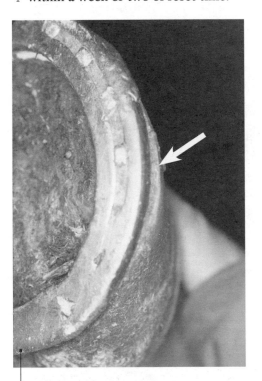

Richard says . . .

MAKE ROOM

I typically leave the edge of the shoe exposed from the middle of the hoof back to the heels equal to the thickness of a dime. Upright hooves can get by with less expansion room because they don't spread much as they grow. Low hooves that tend to flare require more expansion room. Also, hooves in very dry climates don't spread as much as those in wet climates, so desert shoes can be fit closer, with less expansion than swamp shoes.

Past Time for a Reset

If you see that the hoof has become wider than the shoe, it is past time to have the shoes reset. To prevent hoof damage, get your farrier out to your barn as soon as possible. This is especially important if the ground is wet. A hoof weakened by too much moisture can spread out and break down surprisingly fast.

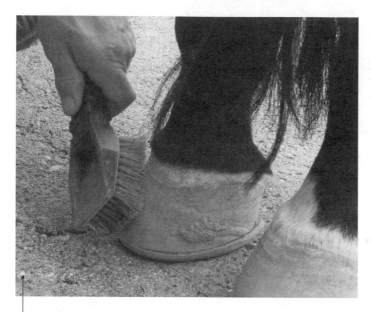

Brush the Hoof Wall
Use a stiff brush to remove dirt and manure from the hoof wall. It is sometimes handy to use the end or edge of the brush to scrape off mud before brushing.

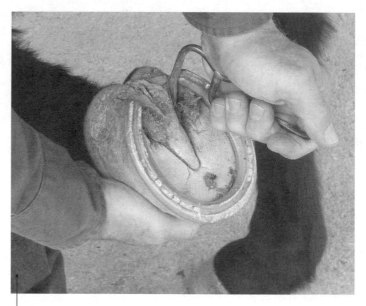

First Pick Away from You
When picking out the sole and clefts of your horse's hooves, use a hoof pick that is comfortable and secure in your hand, and direct the strokes away from your body. This is when you remove the majority of the packed material.

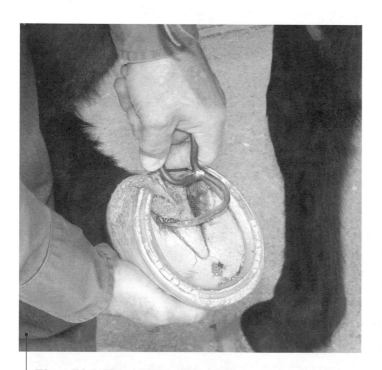

Then Pick Toward You Carefully
Next, turn the hoof pick around and clean out the clefts. As you scrape with the pick, remove all the dirt, but be careful not to dig so deep that you enter sensitive tissue.

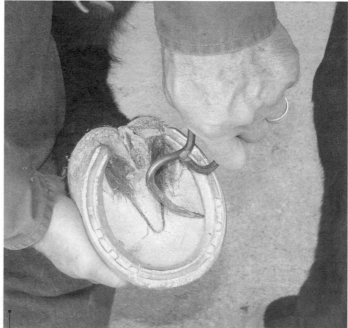

Clean Around Inner Edge of Shoe
Using the tip of the hoof pick, clean around the inside edge of the shoe where it meets the sole.

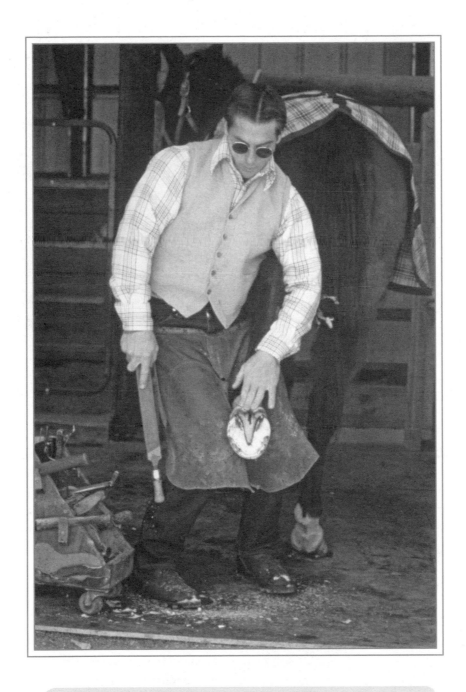

Cherry says . . .

STAY ON SCHEDULE

Finding a good farrier and maintaining a regular hoof-care schedule are two of the most important health-care details a horse owner must manage. Most hoof problems can be avoided by timely farrier visits.

-6-
TACK
AND TOOLS

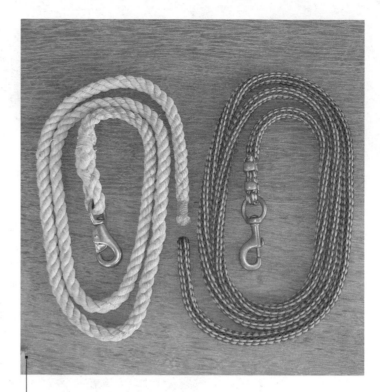

Handling horses is inherently dangerous, and using the wrong tools, or equipment that is in disrepair, is just asking for trouble. Well-made, well-maintained tools and gear will make taking care of your horse's hooves safer, easier, and more effective.

Some tools, like ropes and halters, are used for everyday horse handling. Others, such as shoe pull-offs, are specifically designed for hoof care. Check your everyday and specialized tools and equipment regularly for signs of wear and damage. And be sure to store them properly in a clean, dry place so they'll be ready when you need them.

Cherry says . . .

INVEST IN SAFETY

Good-quality halters and leads might cost more but if properly cared for, they'll outlast three "bargain" items. Safety is one place you don't want to cut cost corners.

Lead Ropes

A lead rope 10 feet (3 m) long and ⅝ inch to ¾ inch (1.6–1.9 cm) in diameter is an appropriate size and length for leading a horse and tying him for trimming and shoeing. A snap securely fastened to one end of the rope should be strong enough not to break if the horse pulls back. It also should be easy to operate with one hand. Solid brass or stainless steel snaps are a good choice. Beware of cheap cast snaps, because they are more likely to break under pressure.

A twisted cotton rope (pictured, on the left) is generally easier on your hands than a rope made of synthetic material, and for this reason, it is often preferred for in-hand work. A drawback to cotton is that it frays and rots more readily than most synthetics and can become hard if it repeatedly gets wet.

Nylon is the most popular material for synthetic ropes. A nylon rope (pictured, on the right) can be almost as soft as cotton, but the close braid typically used for lead ropes makes a smooth surface that can be hard to grip, and it will definitely cause a rope burn if it pulls through your hands. Nylon is much stronger than cotton and resists fraying and rotting. It is a good choice for outdoor tying.

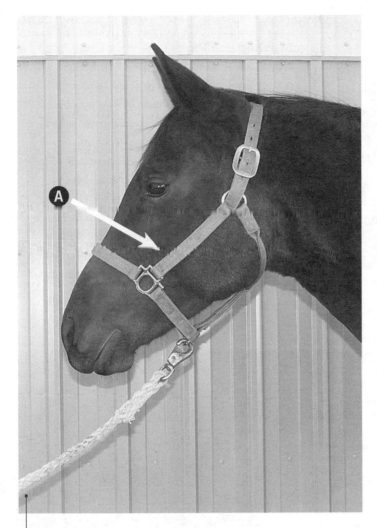

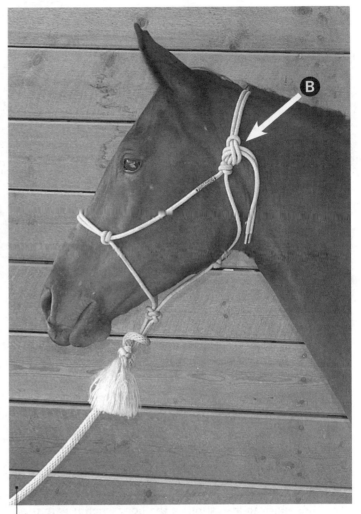

Web Halter

A web halter must fit properly — not too tight or too roomy. The noseband should be positioned two finger-widths below the prominent cheekbone **(A)**. If the halter is too low, it could lie on the fragile tip of the nasal bone, which might become fractured if too much pressure is exerted on the noseband. If the halter is too tight, it can put constant pressure on the horse's poll, nose, and jaw and make the horse uncomfortable. The constant pressure can numb the tissues that come into contact with the tight halter and make the horse unresponsive to cues.

Doubled and stitched nylon web with solid brass hardware and buckles is the best web halter combination. Leather halters are okay for in-hand work but are not strong enough for tying a horse.

Rope Halter

A rope halter fits much like a web halter but is tied with a sheet bend knot **(B)** rather than buckled to fasten. A good rope halter is at least as strong as a good nylon halter, if not stronger. This is because there is no hardware or stitching to break. Many horse trainers prefer a thin rope halter for in-hand work because it elicits a better response from the horse, and thus better control, than does a web halter. If you tie to a hitching post or rail, a rope halter works well. Because a rope halter doesn't have cheek piece hardware the way a web halter does, it is not suitable for cross-ties.

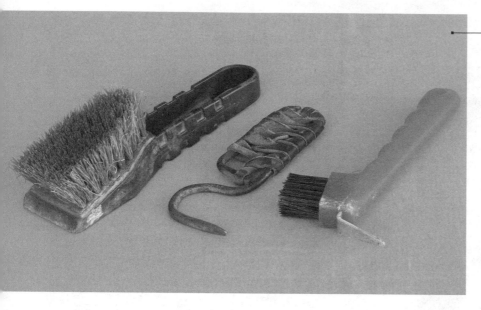

Brushes and Picks

A stiff brush and scraper tool combination is very useful for cleaning dried mud and manure from the hoof wall before you pick up the hoof. A hoof pick should be comfortable for you to hold and easy to handle so that you will not hesitate to use it often. The tip should be long and slender enough to reach to the bottom of the sulci for cleaning but not so sharp or pointed that it will pierce or scratch the tissues. A combo tool with a small, stiff brush and a hoof pick is handy but not as effective as a full-sized brush and well-designed hoof pick.

Hoof Stand

A hoof stand has long been standard equipment for farriers, and many horse owners find this device handy for cleaning and grooming their horse's feet. Traditionally, a hoof stand was used to support the front or hind foot when it was brought forward for hoof work. Today, hoof stands are available with cradles that can also support the hoof when it is in the back position and are an alternative to holding the hoof in one hand or between your knees.

A hoof stand can be a back saver for the occasional hoof handler, but it can also be the cause of injury to you and your horse if he should jerk his leg and tip the stand over. Be sure to invest the time it takes to get your horse used to having each of his hooves on the stand. And always keep one hand on a hoof when it is on a hoof stand, no matter how well trained your horse is.

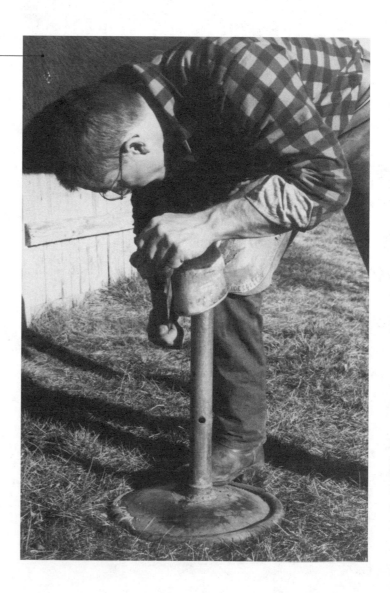

There are a variety of liquid and paste hoof products that protect your horse's hooves from dirt, moisture, urine, manure, ammonia, and other contaminants. Others are available for polishing hooves for the show ring.

HOOF PRODUCTS TO CHOOSE FROM

Hoof sealers are generally clear gels or thin liquids that soak into the hoof to form a barrier against dirt and moisture.

Hoof hardeners or tougheners are designed to make the hoof stronger and more resistant to chipping and cracking. Some of these products rely on a superficial layer of resin or varnish to reinforce the hoof wall. Others contain chemicals that penetrate past the outer wall and change the molecular structure of the keratin that makes up the hoof wall.

Effective sealers and hardeners will not interfere with the way the hoof breathes but will allow the natural moisture from inside the hoof to be released while preventing external moisture from soaking into the hoof. Both types of products can benefit a horse with weak, cracked, or crumbly hooves, as well as one who lives in a very wet or a very dry environment. They are also beneficial when the natural outer coating of the hoof has been worn away or rasped when shaping the hoof during trimming.

Hoof dressings come in paste and liquid varieties and typically contain oils and other ingredients added to soften and even, purportedly, to nourish the hoof. Many hoof dressings make the horse owner feel good about their attentiveness to the care of the horse but don't actually affect the hoof one way or the other. Other dressings can make a hoof too soft if applied often.

Except in the case of very dry heel bulbs (see page 93), a healthy, strong hoof is naturally dry and hard and does not require the application of hoof dressing of any kind.

Hoof polish is like fingernail polish and is used to make hooves look shiny for the show ring. Both clear and black hoof polish are available in oil-based and water-based formulas. Water-based products are easier to remove after a show.

Hoof antiseptics to treat infections are available in liquids, pastes, and creams. Applicators vary from spray and squirt bottles to syringes to brushes. Some products are applied regularly as preventatives while others are designed to treat thrush and other maladies that affect the hooves.

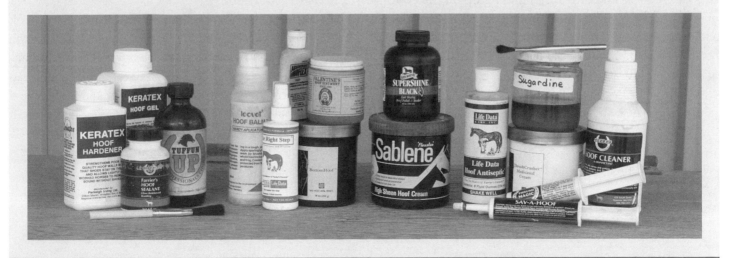

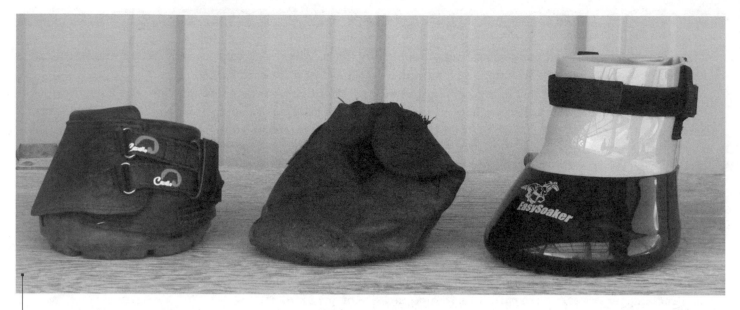

Left to Right: Riding Boot, Emergency Boot, Treatment Boot

HOOF BOOTS

Hoof boots are fitted over the horse's hooves for temporary protection or for medication purposes. There are three general types of hoof boots: riding boots, emergency boots, and treatment boots.

Riding boots are used instead of shoes to protect the hooves when riding or exercising a horse. Some models can also be used over horseshoes for added protection or to prevent snow and dirt from building up on the bottom of shod hooves. Riding hoof boots are more substantial and sturdier than emergency boots, but they vary greatly between brands in how easy (or difficult) they are to put on and take off and how well they stay on and in place without twisting when riding.

Emergency boots are used to protect the hoof until the farrier can replace a lost shoe. A riding hoof boot can also make a fine emergency boot for at-home use, but compact, lightweight emergency boots are more convenient to take along when riding. Unless you find a model that will fit both front and hind hooves, you may need to have two emergency boots at the barn or with you on the trail. An emergency trail boot should fit your horse's foot well so that if you need to travel miles on the trail with one it won't abrade the pastern and coronet. For this reason, many trail riders prefer to take a riding boot along for use as an emergency boot.

Treatment boots are used to protect an injured hoof, keep it clean, and/or hold medication in place against the hoof. They are a welcome replacement for the yards of bandaging material, tape, and wraps used to protect an injured foot. Some treatment boots are watertight and can be filled with water and/or a medication to soak a hoof, say for an abscess. (See page 121.) Other boots are breathable — a better choice for protecting the hoof when the boot is on for more than a few hours at a time.

SHOE REMOVAL KIT

When you need to remove a shoe in an emergency, don't risk injuring your horse or yourself by wrenching off the shoe with a screwdriver and pliers. Having the right tools can make it easy for you to remove a shoe without causing your horse discomfort or damaging his hoof in the process.

Tools for Removing Shoes

You'll need to keep the most basic farrier tools on hand for emergency shoe removal. (See pages 74–78 for the proper use of these tools.)

Hammers of just about any type that weigh between 10 and 16 ounces can be used to strike a clinch cutter effectively.

Clinch cutters don't actually cut the clinches but open them so the straightened nails can slide out easily through the hoof wall as the shoe is pulled.

Rasps have a fine and a coarse side. The fine side is suitable for filing off the clinches instead of opening them with a clinch cutter. There are drawbacks to rasping the clinches, however. (See page 88.)

Crease nail pullers can be a real lifesaver. After you've opened the clinches, you can use the pointed, narrow jaws to fit into the crease of the horseshoe and grab the nail heads. This way you can pull the nails one by one. For most novices, this is much easier than pulling the entire shoe off and is less stressful for the horse.

Pull-offs are used to grab the shoe and pry it off once the clinches are filed off or opened.

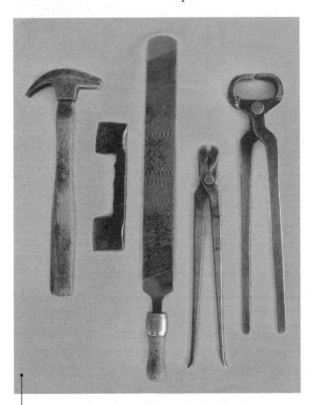

Left to right: Hammer, Clinch Cutter, Rasp, Crease Nail Puller, Pull-off

-7-

BAREFOOT

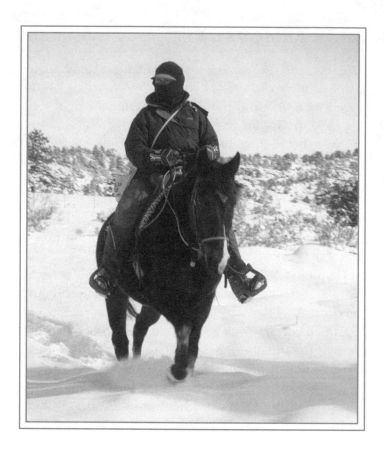

In the current age of natural this, and natural that, the "barefoot bug" has bitten many a horse owner. Some have had trouble with shoes and shoers. Some see barefoot as a way to reduce shoeing and trimming bills or eliminate them altogether by trimming their own horses. Others want their horses to be "natural" and live like wild horses. The reality is that domestic horses by definition are not natural. Riding is not natural. Feeding grain is not natural. Confinement in a stall, pen, or even a pasture is not natural. Don't let your vision of your horse as "wild" override the proven physics and beneficial results of practical farriery. If horseshoes are needed for the well-being of your horse, consider them as natural as baled hay.

Many horses get along fine without horseshoes. Whether or not your horse will remain comfortable and sound barefoot depends on his hoof and limb conformation, the activities he is used for, the environment he lives in, and your level of management.

Most wild (feral, see box) horses' hooves are relatively healthy, in large part because the horses can move freely over a variety of terrain. Natural selection favors individuals with healthy, tough feet; horses with debilitating hoof lameness simply don't survive to breed. Artificial selection imposed by humans, however, often ignores hoof quality altogether and focuses instead on cosmetic traits like coat color or ear shape.

A wild hoof on a wild horse is not necessarily better than a well-managed domestic hoof. In fact, many wild horses survive despite poor feet. By the same token, many barefoot domestic horses are sound and comfortable, while others suffer acute and chronic hoof problems. A barefoot horse that remains sound on pasture or in a pen might not do so well when required to carry the additional weight of tack and rider, especially over varied terrain or at gaits he wouldn't choose on his own.

WILD OR FERAL?

It is now common and generally acceptable to refer to feral horses as wild horses. But biologically speaking, a wild horse is one that has never been domesticated and does not descend from domesticated horses. The last truly wild horses mysteriously disappeared from North America along with saber-toothed cats, mammoths, and most other large mammals around the end of the last ice age, 9 to 13 thousand years ago.

A feral horse is a free-roaming, untamed horse that has descended from domestic horses. North American feral horses are descendants of horses brought to the continent by Spanish conquistadors and others in the 1500s. These herds of feral horses later became known as mustangs and are now commonly called wild horses.

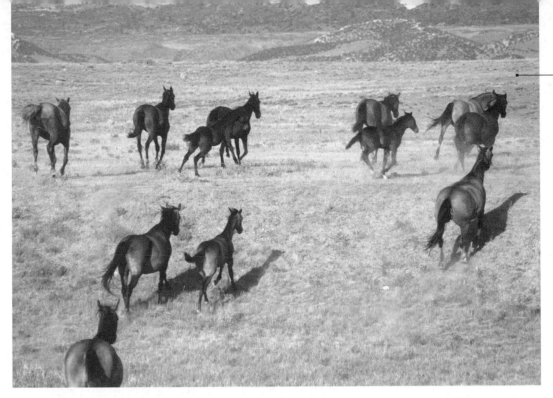

Wild Horses Travel Many Miles Every Day
Wild horses' hooves are conditioned by traveling tens of miles every day over fairly abrasive dry ground. Domestic horses are typically confined to small spaces with soft, often damp footing. A barefoot horse must have sufficient daily exercise to condition the hooves.

TO SHOE OR NOT TO SHOE

After checking with your farrier and vet to see if it's healthy and wise to allow your horse to go barefoot, consider the pros and cons.

Barefoot Advantages

- The owner will have lower-cost farrier visits (trimming costs less than shoeing).
- A properly trimmed bare hoof self-cleans better than a shod hoof.
- A bare hoof can have better traction than a conventionally shod hoof on some terrain, such as rocks or concrete.
- A barefoot horse is safer around humans and other horses should he strike or kick.
- A bare hoof is less likely than a shod hoof to get caught on a fence or halter and cause injury.
- A bare hoof can more readily release excess moisture when it has gotten wet and thus can better maintain optimal moisture equilibrium.

Barefoot Disadvantages

- A bare hoof can wear excessively and break and chip more easily, leading to bruises, abscesses, and lameness.
- A barefoot horse can have higher overall maintenance costs due to the need for more frequent trimming and possible veterinarian and farrier visits required for treating bruises and hoof damage.
- A bare hoof, because of pawing or moving on abrasive ground, can be quickly worn out of balance or can become very short, conditions that can lead to gait defects and lameness.
- A barefoot horse may lack confidence on rough or stony ground because of sole pressure and sensitivity.
- A bare hoof has less traction on some surfaces and for some activities than a hoof shod specifically for those surfaces or activities.
- If hoof boots are needed to protect bare hooves for riding or exercise, it takes longer to get the horse ready.

SHOULD YOU PULL SHOES FOR WINTER?

During the era of horse-powered agriculture, it became a common practice to pull the shoes off draft horses that weren't working and turn these animals out for the winter. Turning a shod horse out in a snow-covered cornfield, plowed field, or winter pasture would have been an open invitation for lost shoes and damaged hooves. And shod horses turned out and fed in a group are more likely to injure one another should they kick.

Today, pulling the shoes for part of the year is still a popular practice, and it works well for some horses, but for others it can lead to temporary or long-term hoof problems. The money you save by not shoeing during the winter might result in double the expense for hoof repair come spring.

Bare hooves are most vulnerable right after the shoes are pulled. A hoof wall weakened by nail holes is more likely to chip and break when no longer protected by a shoe. Soles that have been elevated and protected by shoes are susceptible to bruising by stones and hard ground when bared. It takes between six weeks and six months for nail holes to grow out and for hooves to become conditioned to going barefoot. Horses living in a wet environment and those getting insufficient exercise or improper trimming may never develop hooves that will do well barefoot.

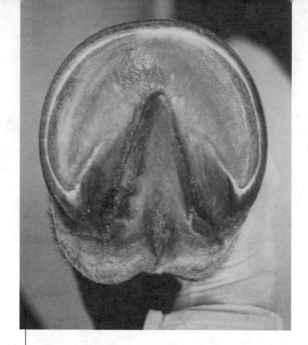

Good Bare Hoof Candidate
A good candidate for going barefoot has high-quality hoof material: thick, dense, hard, and solid, yet resilient because of a proper balance between internal and external moisture. The hoof wall is thick and solid through the quarters and into the heel. The bottom of the hoof is well cupped with a durable, resilient, concave sole. The sole is thick and hard enough that the horse can walk on gravel without showing signs of discomfort.

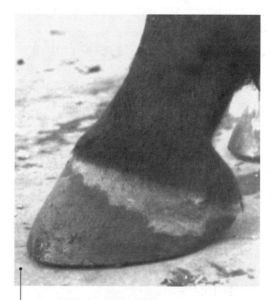

Good Bare Hoof Angle
A barefoot candidate has a normal upright hoof and pastern axis of 54 degrees or greater. The heel angle is parallel to the toe angle. The hoof is free of dishes or flares; the wall is straight from the coronary band to the ground. With proper management, some hooves that at first appear to be poor barefoot candidates can be conditioned and reshaped into healthy, sound bare hooves.

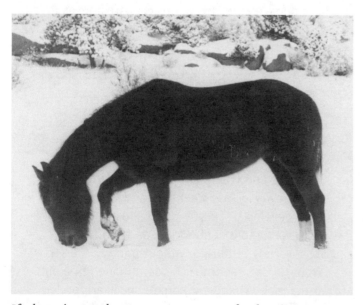

If a horse is turned out on a snowy pasture for the winter, barefoot is ideal.

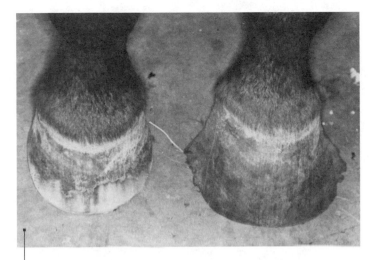

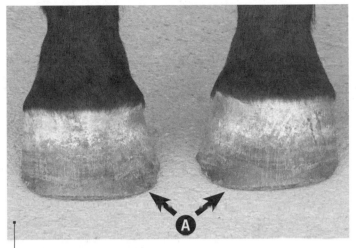

What a Difference a Trim Makes

Some hooves need to be trimmed before they can be evaluated. This horse was kept in a wet pen, and his feet were neglected. This caused his hooves to flare out and begin to break off at the quarters. Once the hooves were trimmed, however, it became apparent that they were of good quality. If kept in a dry environment and trimmed every three to five weeks, he could go barefoot during free time without problems. Depending on how his hooves toughen up, he may or may not need to wear hoof boots or shoes for riding and exercising.

Imbalance from Pawing

A horse's behavior may cause his hooves to wear down so short or become so imbalanced that they require shoes to prevent lameness. For example, this horse has the habit of pawing, which consistently wears the front toes low on the outside and creates a point **(A)** on the inside. Frequent rasping could keep the hooves balanced, but they then might become too short for comfort. Shoes can keep the hooves balanced and the horse comfortable and sound.

Weaving, pacing, stall walking, and kicking are examples of other behaviors that cause horses' hooves to become imbalanced.

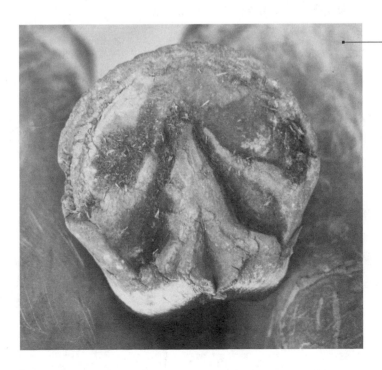

Excess Length Leads to Broken Hooves

It's a common misconception that bare hooves need less-frequent care than do shod hooves. In fact, keeping a bare hoof in top shape often requires more frequent trimming. An optimal interval for shoeing is five to eight weeks. An optimal interval for trimming bare hooves is more like three to five weeks.

Bare hooves need lots of exercise on abrasive ground in order to condition hoof tissues and wear down the hooves sufficiently to match growth. A hoof that is allowed to grow too long, like the one shown here, will begin cracking and breaking out in pieces, often starting at the quarters.

A GOOD TRIM BY ANY OTHER NAME

When I was learning the farrier trade, there were two kinds of hoof trims: good and bad. Good trims had balanced hooves and rounded edges to minimize flares and chipping; at the farrier's discretion, the quarters might be sculpted out some and the toe squared a bit. Six weeks later, the hoof still looked good, just longer. Bad trims typically had low heels, long toes, and sharp edges. A bad trim looked bad from the outset.

Today there is a veritable smorgasbord of trims on the market with names like barefoot trim, pasture trim, natural trim, four-point trim, and natural-balance trim. Most of these methods stem from observations of healthy feral-horse hooves. Some hoof-care practitioners stress marketing catchwords and gimmicks more than practical results. A good trim, no matter what it's called, is one that keeps your horse sound for his intended purpose.

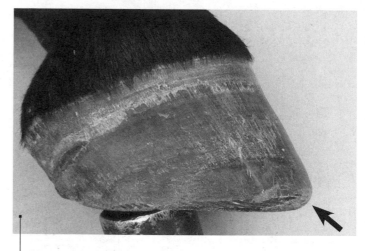

Mustang Roll

When a hoof is trimmed for shoeing, the bottom edge is left sharp to allow the hoof wall to have maximum contact with the horseshoe. Without the protection of a shoe, a hoof trimmed like this would immediately begin breaking and chipping along the bottom edge and would be susceptible to splitting and cracks.

When a hoof is trimmed for going barefoot, the edges of the hoof should be rounded or beveled, all around the hoof, to at least half the thickness of the hoof wall (see arrow). This makes it easier for the hoof to break over in any direction and minimizes flaring, chipping, and cracking of the hoof wall. This rounding of the hoof perimeter is sometimes called a "mustang roll" after the shape of wild horses' hooves.

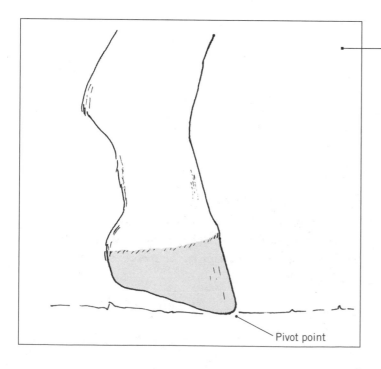

Pivot point

Breakover

Breakover is the pivoting movement of a hoof at the toe from the time the heels lift up until the toe leaves the ground. The hoof is a lever with the toe as the fulcrum or pivot point. The pull of the flexor tendons is the force that lifts the heels and rotates the hoof over the toe. The longer the toe of the hoof, the farther the force is from the fulcrum and the more force it takes to lift the heels. A long toe makes it harder for the hoof to break over and puts more stress on the structures of the hoof. (See page 126.)

FOAL TRIMMING

A foal will usually be somewhat knock-kneed until six or eight months of age, depending on chest conformation. The more narrow the chest, the more the face of the knee will naturally (and should be allowed to) rotate out to the side. The fetlocks also face somewhat outward to allow horizontal formation and maintenance of the growth plates. At eight to ten months of age, the normal widening of the foal's chest allows the knees and fetlocks to straighten up and rotate inward so that they are more directly situated under the body mass and line up in a straight column.

Improper "corrective" trimming of a foal to force the fetlocks and hoof to face forward can damage the fetlock and result in a toed-in stance when the foal matures. Foals that have genetics for heavy bodies and wide chests definitely should not be trimmed early or aggressively for their knock-kneed, toed-out condition, or by the time their chests widen, they may become bowlegged.

If kept level and balanced through his growing months, the foal that has mild to moderate knock-knees will stand relatively straight as a yearling.

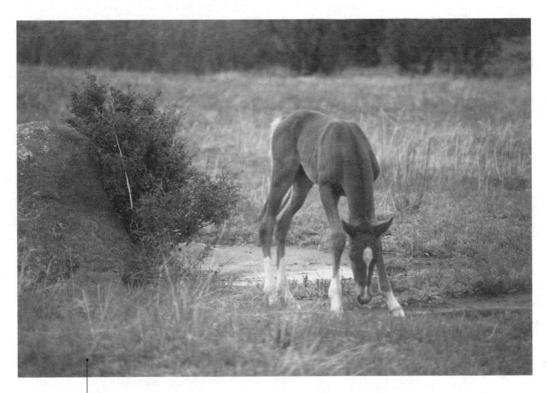

Short Neck, Long Legs: Where's the Grass?
Because a newborn foal's legs are longer than his neck, he has to use an adaptive stance to eat near the ground. To stabilize himself and to reach the ground for grazing, the foal widens his base of support by spreading his front legs. This rotates the lower leg outward and brings the knees close together, making the foal appear knock-kneed.

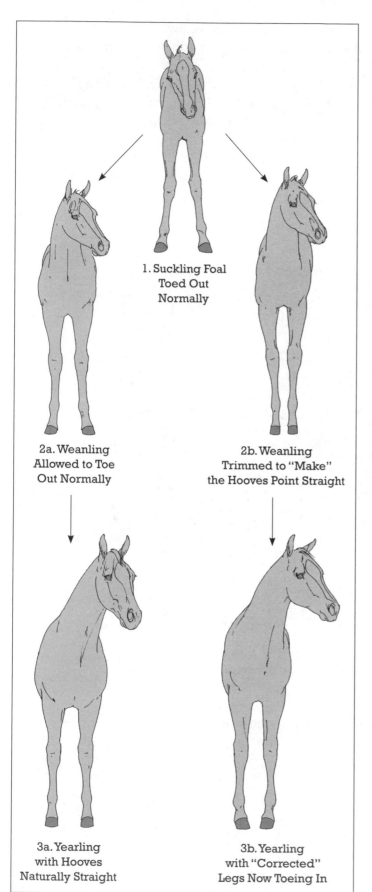

1. Suckling Foal
Toed Out
Normally

2a. Weanling
Allowed to Toe
Out Normally

2b. Weanling
Trimmed to "Make"
the Hooves Point Straight

3a. Yearling
with Hooves
Naturally Straight

3b. Yearling
with "Corrected"
Legs Now Toeing In

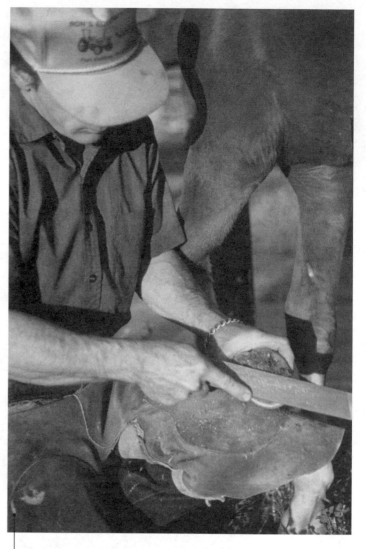

Foal Trimming Schedule

A farrier experienced in foal trimming will assess the balance of your foal's hooves in relation to his limbs and hoof-wear patterns. He can then determine how often the foal needs hoof care. Rasping required to balance a foal's hoof is done conservatively and as often as necessary. Some foals may need rasping every week or so while others might go four or five weeks between farrier visits.

BOOTS FOR BARE HOOVES

Hoof boots have evolved in design and materials to the degree that they can be a practical alternative to shoes. Appropriate boots will protect a horse's hooves when he is being ridden or exercised, but it is important that you take the boots off when the horse is not in use. Leaving hoof boots on for extended periods can cause rubbing, chafing, and moisture buildup from hoof respiration, which can lead to weak hooves and bacterial and fungal infections.

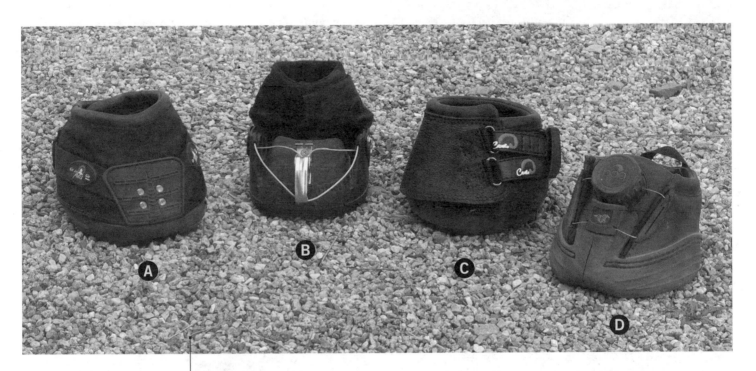

Riding Boots

Boots designed for riding or for exercise are typically fastened by Velcro straps **(A, C)** or by some sort of cable tensioning system **(B, D).** Horses' feet vary greatly in size and shape, and it's important to take the time to find a size and model of hoof boot that fits securely and snugly enough to stay in place without rubbing on the sensitive areas of the foot, specifically the bulbs of the heels, coronary band, and pastern.

Each manufacturer has specific guidelines for measuring the hooves to get the proper size, and most manufacturers allow you to return or exchange boots that don't fit — as long as they are in new condition. Therefore, when you first try the boots on your horse, take care that his hooves and the surface he is standing on are very clean and dry.

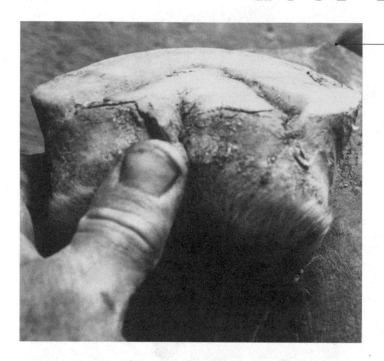

Hoof-Boot Candidates

Boots can be used to protect hooves that are making the transition from being shod to going barefoot. Hooves with very short walls and a flat sole, for example, can use boots during work to prevent wear on the wall so it can grow longer more quickly. A horse with very thin or soft soles or hooves that are worn very short might continue to be footsore even with the use of boots. To help in the meantime, you could use soft cushion inserts that are available with some boots. These insoles can help make a sensitive horse more comfortable while working. Once his hooves grow down, toughen up, and become less sensitive, the inserts will no longer be necessary.

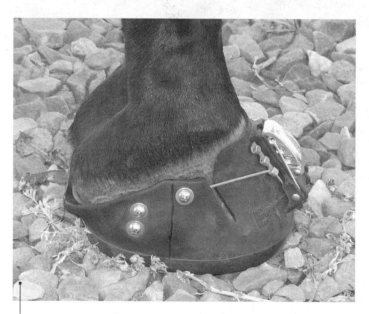

Low Rider Boot

A hoof boot that fits below the coronet will be less likely to cause rubbing or chafing of skin areas. However, a low-fitting boot is less secure than a boot that extends to the pastern and is more likely to come off the hoof while in use.

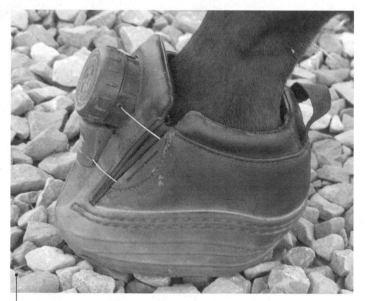

High-Rise Boot

A hoof boot that extends above the coronary band is more likely to stay on the horse's hoof, but depending on the design and how well it fits, it could rub and chafe the coronet, pastern, or heel bulbs. Take care when choosing and applying boots of this type to make sure they fit properly. Then check the horse's feet often, especially the pastern area, when using the boots, to make sure they are tightened properly and are not causing problems.

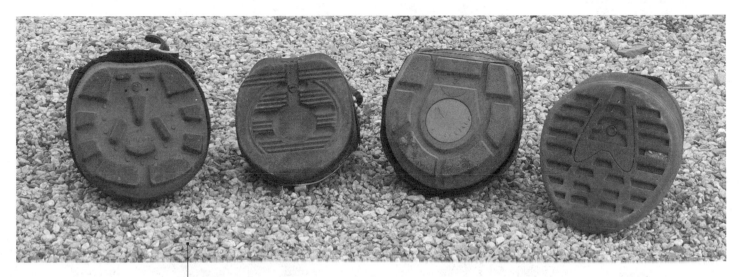

Boot Traction

Like tires, hoof boots have different traction patterns, and the larger the tread and more aggressive the traction, the faster the wear. Less-distinct tread with lesser traction usually wears longer. Too little traction can cause a horse to slip, especially on wet grass, pavement, or ice. Too much traction can prevent the foot from sliding or twisting naturally on the ground in the manner of a bare or normally shod hoof. This excess grab can cause joint injuries.

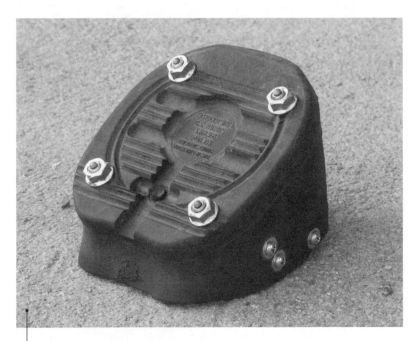

Boot Studs for Traction

Some hoof-boot models are designed to accept screw-in studs for increased traction when riding on snow, ice, and frozen or soft wet ground.

Drains and Gaiters

Most hoof boots have small holes (drains) in the bottom so that any water that gets inside the boot, as will happen when crossing a puddle or stream, can drain out. Gaiters are like short neoprene socks that are used with riding hoof boots to prevent mud and other debris from getting into the boots. Gaiters can also prevent or minimize chafing and help secure the boots on the hooves (some horse owners use sections of sheer nylon stockings to prevent chafing). Gaiters are an integral part of some riding hoof boots and are also available separately.

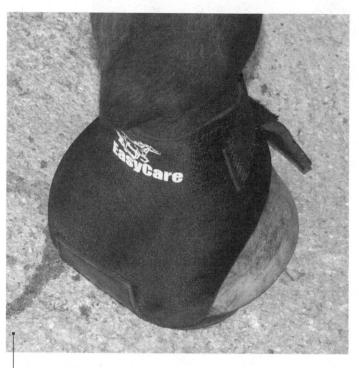

Separate Gaiter

A gaiter that is purchased separately from the hoof boot is applied to the pastern before the boot is put on the hoof as shown above. This type of gaiter is typically connected to a thin pad that slides under the hoof inside the boot to keep the gaiter from riding up.

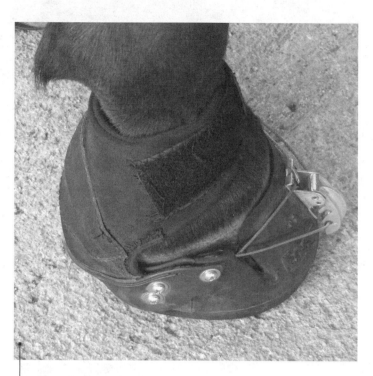

Integral Gaiter

A gaiter that is part of the boot greatly reduces the risk that the boot will come off without your making efforts to remove it.

Richard says . . .

PREVENT BOOT BUILDUP

When using hoof boots, always be aware of the type of ground you are riding over and pay attention to how your horse is behaving and moving. Sand, gravel, and mud can accumulate inside a boot and put pressure on the sole and frog, causing the horse discomfort, especially with boots not fitted with gaiters. If your horse is suddenly reluctant to move forward or begins to stumble, dismount and remove each boot to check for debris.

-8-
HORSESHOES, AND WHY

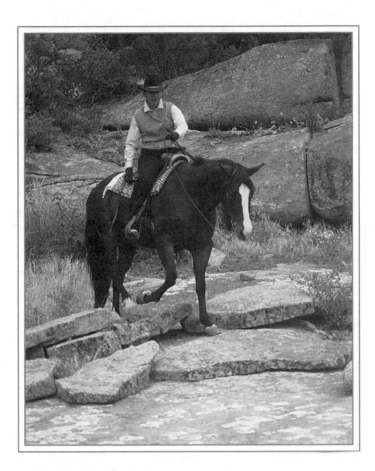

When horses were first domesticated about 4000 BCE, they began to experience a number of lifestyle changes that negatively affected hoof quality and condition. Most notable was the change in mobility. Wild horses were nomads — wandering from place to place, seeking feed, shelter, and safety. These native horses evolved on semi-arid plains but when domesticated, they were moved to stalls, pens, and pastures that were often wet. Rather than wandering, they suddenly had limited, controlled exercise. Confinement also brought about a dramatic dietary shift from free-range native prairie grass to once- or twice-a-day feedings of grains and cultivated hays, including alfalfa.

Wild horses survived by their strength, speed, and agility, and by their natural ability to avoid injury. Natural selection allowed the strongest to survive and thrive. With domestication came man's care, but also his selection criteria. Tough, durable hooves were not always a priority. In fact, at times, very small hooves have been in vogue. Throughout the ages, breeders have selected for color, coat patterns, and other cosmetic traits over hoof soundness.

To keep horses sound and useful, man has tried various means of protecting a horse's feet over the millennia, everything from grass, to wood, to rawhide. Eventually, around the fifth century CE, nails were used to attach iron horseshoes. This method of protection proved to be economical and effective and has been used ever since.

TYPES OF HOOF CARE

Whether or not your horse needs shoes depends on his hoof and limb conformation, his intended use, and your management. All domestic horses require regular trimming.

Preventive hoof care, sometimes called natural hoof care, is characterized by trimming and shoeing for balance, support, and protection. The goals of preventive hoof care are long-term soundness and performance longevity, which are achieved by circumventing hoof problems through regular maintenance. Preventive principles should be the basis of every horse's routine hoof-care program.

Corrective trimming and shoeing consists of altering the hoof shape and balance or using specialized shoes, or both, to affect a horse's stance or movement.

Therapeutic shoeing is often a part of a lameness treatment designed to protect and support a damaged hoof or limb or to prevent or encourage a particular movement until healing can take place. Therapeutic farriery can be essential to the treatment of some kinds of lameness, but other kinds will gain no benefit from shoeing.

Vanity shoeing includes the use of weighted shoes or excessively long feet on gaited horses to exaggerate leg action and to build up show feet on draft horses to make hooves appear larger than they are.

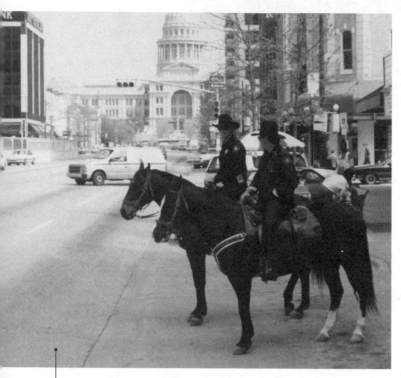

Shoes Prevent Excessive Wear

When ridden on abrasive terrain such as pavement, a horse's hooves can quickly wear out of balance or become dangerously short. Shoes prevent hoof wear and maintain hoof balance, thereby enabling the horse to function comfortably and remain sound.

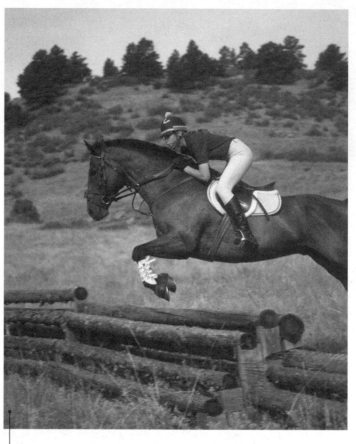

Shoes Provide Support

Properly applied shoes can optimize the support of the limb and help stabilize the hoof during extreme stress, such as landing after jumping.

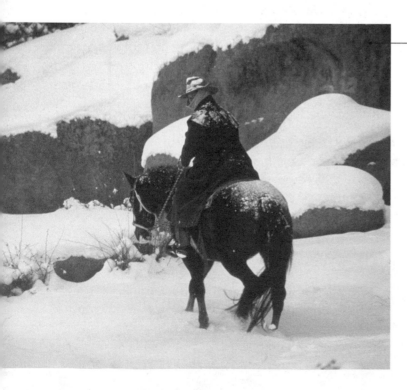

Shoes Provide Traction

To perform safely, confidently, and without unnecessary exertion, a horse needs traction that is appropriate for the footing and for the activity. If a horse needs greater traction than would be provided by a plain shoe, traction devices or more aggressive shoes can be used to:

- Increase horse and rider safety.
- Increase a horse's feeling of security so that he will stride normally.
- Help a horse maintain his balance on unstable footing such as mud, ice, snow, or rock.
- Minimize fatigue.
- Reduce the risk of injury.

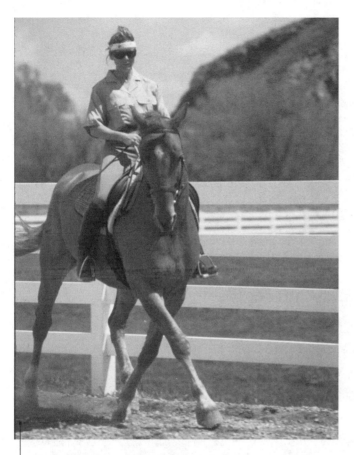

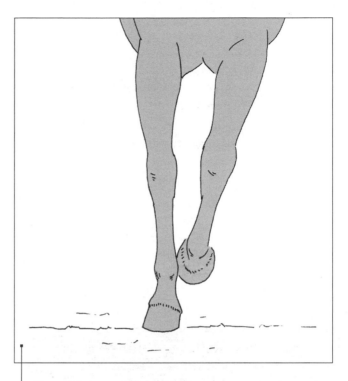

Shoes Correct Gait Problems

Gait abnormalities that cause inefficient movement or interference can be minimized or corrected with the application of properly designed and applied shoes.

Shoes Increase Confidence

It is not uncommon to see horses with good-quality hooves competing barefoot in dressage events working on level, soft footing. However, competitors can never be sure what the footing will be at shows. That's why many keep their horses shod; they know that if a horse slips or steps on a stone, his confidence can be shaken for a while. If arena footing contains gravel, rocks, or uneven ground, shoes can enable the horse to perform at his best.

Cherry says . . .

SHOES BUILD CONFIDENCE

Whether I'm riding in my arena or on a Rocky Mountain trail, I don't want my horse to be tentative in his movement. I want him to be confident and bold. Horseshoes help him have that confidence.

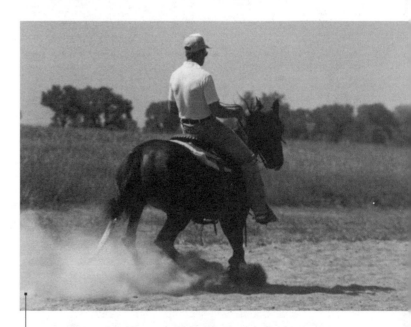

Shoes Can Minimize Traction

In a few instances, the goal is to limit traction. Sliding plates — wide, smooth horseshoes on the hinds that maximize support and minimize traction — enhance some horse maneuvers, such as the dazzling spin and the sliding stop performed in reining classes.

Shoes Prevent Bruising

When the sole is soft or sensitive, or if the horse is going to be used on rocky or rough terrain, full pads between the shoe and the hoof can protect the sole and frog from injury and make the horse more comfortable and confident.

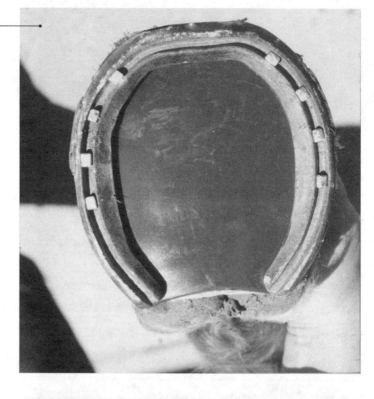

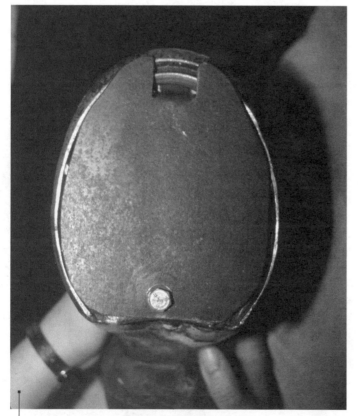

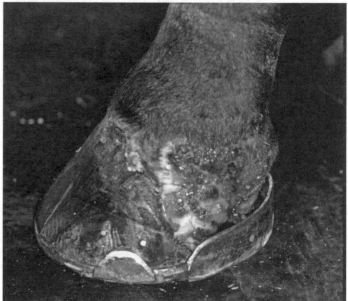

Shoes Offer Protection plus Access

Treatment of injuries to the sole and frog can be made easier by the use of appropriate shoes. A sole abscess, for example, requires cleanliness and complete protection from pressure, yet also must be monitored and treated regularly. A treatment-plate shoe has a removable steel plate that covers the bottom — just what the doctor ordered.

Shoes Provide Medical Support

Treating problems such as laminitis, navicular disease syndrome, underrun heels, and fractured coffin bones is often fruitless without the support that a shoe provides. In the case of a serious crack or other hoof injury that requires removal of a portion of the hoof wall, a specialized shoe can offer support and protection while the hoof heals.

HORSESHOE ANATOMY

Most horseshoes are made of steel, which is a combination of iron, carbon, and other elements. Steel is graded by the amount of carbon it contains; the higher the carbon content, the harder the steel. **Mild steel** (low carbon) is used for horseshoes because it is easily shaped, yet durable enough to last for one or more shoeing periods. All but the largest sizes of mild steel horseshoes can be shaped to fit a hoof without heating the steel to shape it. Large shoes, like those used for warmbloods and draft horses, must be heated in a forge in order to be shaped.

While some farriers prefer to make all or some of the shoes they apply, the vast majority of horseshoes are factory-made "keg shoes," so called because they were once shipped in wooden kegs

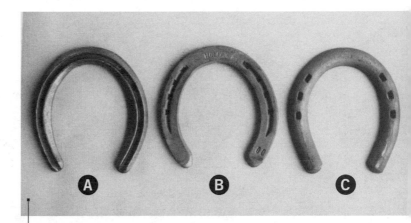

Three Types of Horseshoe Ground Surfaces
A **rim shoe (A)** has a deep crease down the center of the entire ground surface that forms two rims for added traction. A **plain horseshoe (B)** has a crease on each branch extending slightly past the first and last nail holes. A **stamped shoe (C)** has no crease; instead, the nail holes are enlarged at the top to recess the nail heads.

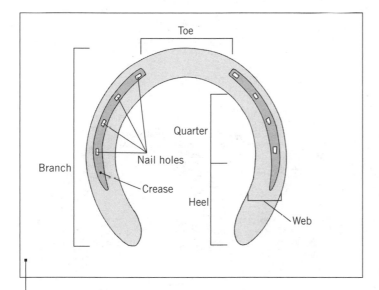

Parts of a Horseshoe

Toe — center front of the shoe between the first two nail holes

Branch — one half of a shoe, from the toe to the heel

Quarter — part of a branch between the first and last nail holes

Heel — part of the branch, from the last nail hole to the end

Nail Holes — rectangular holes to match the size and shape of the shank of a horseshoe nail just below the nail head

Crease or Swedge — a groove in the center of the ground surface into which the heads of the nails are set to protect them from wear

---

Cherry says . . .

RIM SHOES FOR TRACTION

Most of the time, all that Aria or Seeker needs for good traction are rim shoes. Once when I was riding with a friend whose horse was shod with regular shoes, we had to cross a large granite outcropping. Within a few steps, Sue's horse was skating with each foot going in a different direction. Her horse panicked and it was only Sue's great balance and cool head that got them safely across the rock slabs.

My horse, Zinger, had rim shoes, which provided just enough grip and security for us to walk confidently across the rock and wait for our shaky friends on the other side.

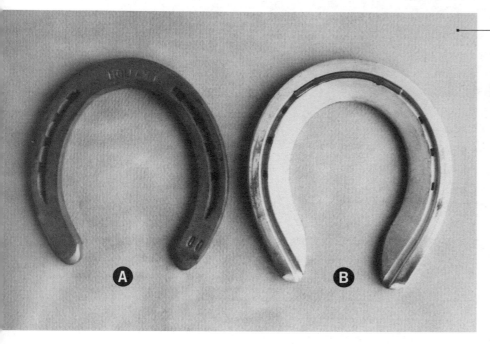

Wide Web Shoes

Wide web shoes available in both steel (**A**) and aluminum (**B**) provide a larger base of support for the foot and protect more of the sole. Because aluminum is lighter than steel, it is used for most racing shoes, which are called plates. Aluminum wears away more quickly than steel, so many aluminum shoes have a steel insert at the toe where most of the wear occurs, to make the shoe last longer. Aluminum shoes also bend more easily than steel shoes and often cannot provide the support a horse needs. This is especially true of larger horses or with jumpers who place a great deal of force on their shoes when landing and turning.

Bar Shoes

A bar shoe has the heels joined and is used to provide additional support to the hoof and leg. There are many creative and functional ways to join the heels of a shoe and as many names to describe the shoes. Below are the four most common bar shoes:

Straight bar shoes (A) have a bar going straight across between the heels.

Egg bar shoes (B) have a curved bar, making the shoe oval, like an egg.

Heart bar shoes (C) have a V-shaped bar that touches and supports the frog.

Full support shoes (D) have a combination of an egg bar and a heart bar.

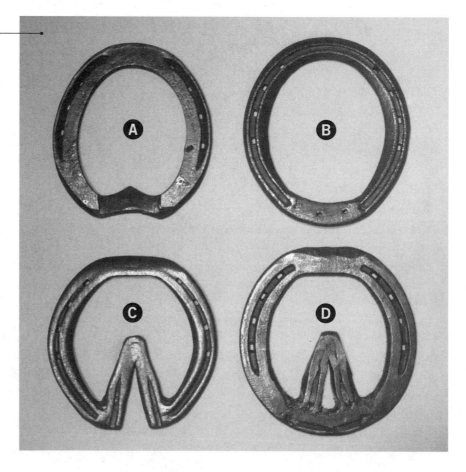

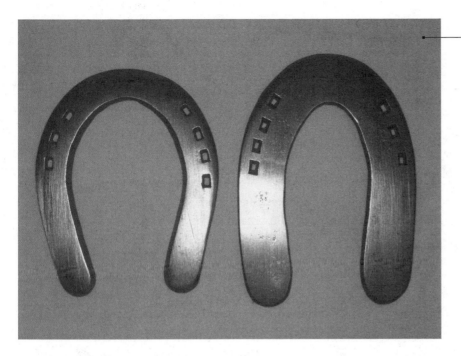

Sliding Plates

Sliding plates enable a reining horse to slide to a stop on his hind feet and to swivel on his hindquarters. Sliding plates are wide, smooth shoes with extended heels and with nail heads that are recessed so they're flush with the ground surface of the shoe. This minimizes traction. Narrow sliders (left) are generally used when first starting to train a reining horse, and as he gains confidence with his reduced traction behind, he graduates to wider sliders (right).

Modified Toes

Modified toe shoes are used to enhance breakover and make it easier for the hoof to pivot over the toe (see page 126). There are basically three ways of modifying the toe:

A **rolled toe** is rounded or beveled on the ground surface of the shoe at the toe, much like the toe of a well-worn horseshoe. The hoof surface of a rolled-toe shoe remains flat, making it easier to fit to a hoof than a rocker-toe shoe.

A **rocker toe** is bent upward. The toe of the hoof must be rasped to match the toe of the shoe so that it fits evenly against the entire bottom of the hoof wall.

A **squared toe** is shaped straight across the toe rather than being rounded in front like a standard horseshoe. The portion of the hoof that extends over the squared toe of the shoe is rasped to prevent it from chipping. (See **C** & **D** on page 62 and drawing on page 117.)

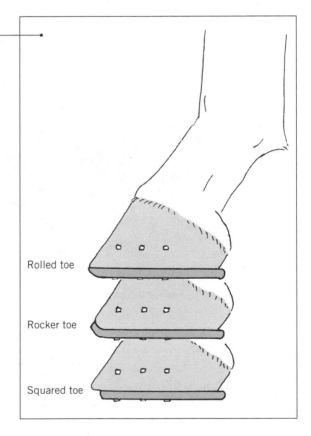

Rolled toe

Rocker toe

Squared toe

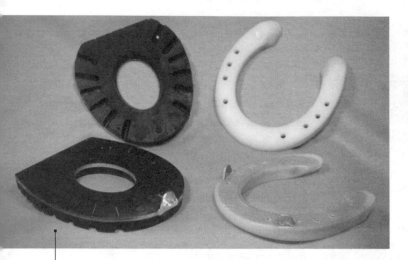

Synthetic Shoes

Synthetic horseshoes are made of flexible rubber and plastic materials, many of which are lighter than steel shoes yet wear just as long. Some shoes have an aluminum core to make the shoes rigid for better support. On most surfaces, synthetic shoes typically provide less traction than do bare hooves or steel shoes. They also can become hard and slippery in cold temperatures.

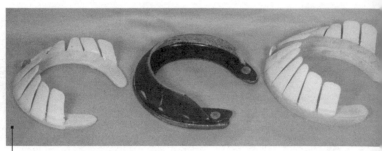

Tab Glue-on Shoes

When a horse's foot is either too sore or in too poor a condition to attach shoes with nails, glue-on shoes are useful. They are also used to correct limb abnormalities in foals, whose hooves are too tiny for safe nailing. Tab-type glue-on shoes are synthetic and typically have an aluminum core. The shoe is shaped to fit the foot using a hammer and anvil, and then each tab is glued to the hoof wall with an instant adhesive. The synthetic cuff in the center of the photo has no metal core but is riveted to a steel shoe that has already been fit to the hoof. Then the cuff with shoe attached is glued to the hoof wall.

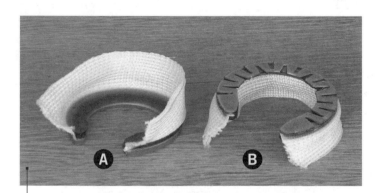

Flexible-Cuff Glue-on Shoes

There are two types of flexible-cuff glue-on shoes. One type consists of an aluminum shoe that comes permanently bonded to a tough fabric cuff (A). The farrier shapes the shoe (with the cuff attached) just like a normal shoe to fit the hoof and then glues the shoe/cuff to the hoof. The second variety is used with a conventional metal horseshoe. It consists of a flexible base that is permanently bonded to a tough fabric cuff (B). The base can be easily bent by hand to match the shape of a horseshoe that has been shaped to fit the hoof. The base is glued to the shoe in one operation, and then the entire cuff assembly is glued to the hoof.

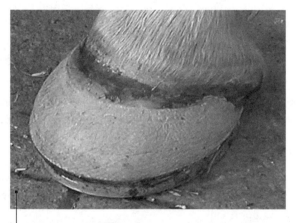

Flexible Cuff Applied

Flexible-cuff shoes are glued to the hoof using acrylic adhesive, which often makes them more secure than shoes that are nailed. They can be used for all types of riding in any environment. However, this option is labor intensive and more expensive than standard shoeing practices. Horse owners typically use the flexible cuffs for horses with sensitive feet that can't tolerate nailing or for poor hooves that won't hold nails.

PADS

Pads are applied between the shoe and the hoof for added sole protection, for shock absorption, or to adjust the hoof angle. A pad is typically made of leather or plastic, and it covers all or part of the sole and frog.

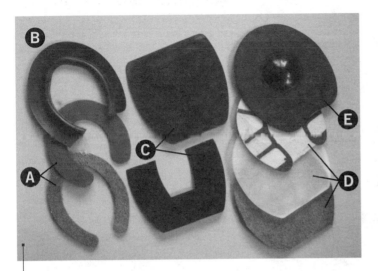

Types of Pads and Their Uses

Rim pads (A) leave the sole and frog open. They are used mainly for shock absorption.

Tube-type rim pads (B) are used to prevent snow buildup on the bottom of a shod hoof. Each pad has a small rubber tube that lines the inside rim of a shoe and is held in place by an attached flat, thin tab (flange) that lies between the shoe and the hoof (see page 70).

Wedge pads (C) are generally used to raise the heels of a low-heeled hoof to bring it into balance. They are available as a bar pad or a full pad.

Full flat pads (D) cover the entire sole. They are used to protect the sole and to keep it clean. Some have varying degrees of shock absorption.

Bubble pads (E) have a dome molded into the center of the ground surface that is designed to keep snow and other icy materials from accumulating next to the sole (snowballing). With full pads, and especially with bubble pads, traction is reduced (see page 70).

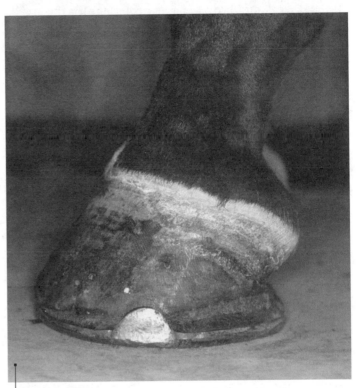

Wedge Pad

Wedge pads are also called degree pads because they are manufactured in various thicknesses to raise a horse's hoof angle from 2 to 6 degrees. They are often used to treat navicular syndrome when the horse has low, underrun heels. Thick wedge pads are also stiff enough to protect the frog and underlying navicular area from direct ground pressure.

HOOF PACKING

Just as you respire through your skin, a hoof releases moisture through the sole and frog. One drawback to using full pads is that they interfere with this normal horse hoof respiration.

A full pad doesn't allow the hoof to breathe, so moisture is trapped against the sole. This can make the sole soft and weak and provide an environment for the smelly growth of bacteria, fungus, and yeast that can harm the hoof. Another problem is that sand, mud, water, and snow can get in between the pad and sole and put pressure on the sole, making the horse uncomfortable and even lame.

The space between the pad and the hoof is usually packed with some type of material to keep foreign matter out and keep the sole healthy. Silicone caulking is a common choice. Typically, silicone is squirted into the sole space using a caulking gun after the shoe and pad are in place. However, silicone does a poor job of keeping sand and mud from accumulating between the pad and sole. And because silicone is totally nonbreathable, moisture and heat are concentrated against the sole. Recently, chemicals such as copper sulfate have been added to commercial silicone packing to minimize bacterial growth.

Some new hoof packing formulations use a rubberlike material that is applied as a thick liquid over a clean, dry sole. This material sets in minutes and adheres to the sole to form a flexible pad. Some of the "pour-on" pads can be used on bare, unshod hooves.

Richard says . . .

CVP DOES THE TRICK

CVP is a hoof packing that I developed in 1984 when I was doing therapeutic farriery for Colorado State University Veterinary Teaching Hospital. CVP stands for three ingredients: copper sulfate, Venice turpentine, and polypropylene hoof felt. Poly felt, which does not readily absorb water, was developed specifically for hoof packing. Copper sulfate is a compound used in agriculture to control fungi, bacteria, and yeast. Venice turpentine is a thick resin from the larch tree. When copper sulfate and Venice turpentine are combined, they form a medicated adhesive that controls the growth of undesirable organisms and binds the poly felt to the sole, forming a protective gasket between the pad and the hoof (see Resource Guide, page 148).

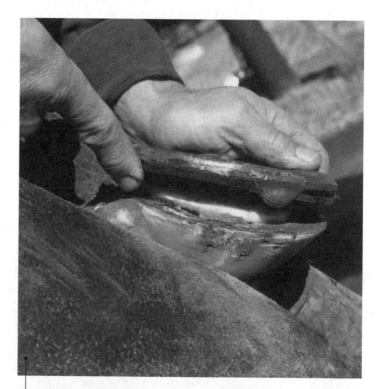

CVP Gasket Pad
The CVP gasket prevents sand, dirt, mud, and other foreign material from getting under the pad. It eliminates the foul odor often associated with the use of other packing and has been useful in treating severe cases of thrush and white line disease.

CLIPS

A clip is a vertical extension of a horseshoe that helps secure a horseshoe on the hoof. Clips can be forged right from a hot shoe, or separate clips can be brazed or welded to the shoe. Horses that have good-quality hooves and that are only moderately active may never need clips because six nails will usually hold a shoe tight for six to eight weeks.

Weak, deteriorated hoof walls that have difficulty holding nails are prime candidates for clips. So are active horses that speed up, turn quickly, jump, or stop hard. Extreme twisting and shearing forces on a shoe can cause the nails to loosen and the shoe to shift on the hoof or come off altogether. Horses that have traction devices such as calks on their shoes can always use the added security that clips provide.

Clips are also used to minimize hoof movement when treating some injuries and following surgeries. With a severe hoof crack, for example, clips help stabilize the hoof until the crack grows out. If a portion of hoof wall must be removed (resected), and the nailing area is therefore limited, clips help secure the shoe until the hoof heals.

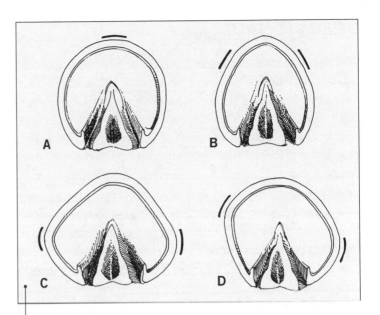

Clip Positions
Clips can be used in various locations to accomplish different goals.

A. A toe clip keeps the shoe from sliding back on the hoof.

B. Side clips near the toe keep the shoe from sliding back and to the side.

C. Quarter clips are used to contain flares at the quarters of the hoof.

D. Asymmetric side clips placed across the widest part of a deformed hoof help the hoof grow into a more balanced, healthy shape.

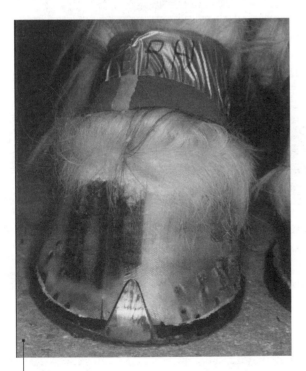

Toe Clip
To keep the shoe from sliding back on the hoof, a single clip can be added at the toe. Clips are often used on draft horses to counteract the force of the heavy shoes hitting the ground with each step and on the front hooves of hunters and jumpers to counteract the impact of landing.

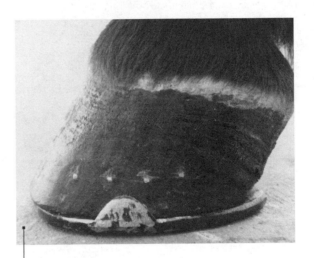

Side Clips
Side clips are commonly installed symmetrically between the first and second or second and third nail holes from the toe. These clip locations prevent the shoe from moving back on the hoof or to either side.

TRACTION

Plain steel shoes, whether creased or stamped, provide adequate traction for most situations. Rim shoes provide added traction because the rims cut into the ground until they are worn down. Also, dirt that packs into the crease on the bottom of a rim shoe provides added traction against the ground. Aluminum shoes have a slightly better grab than steel shoes because aluminum is softer and "grippier."

Traction devices such as calks and ice nails can be added to shoes but they will require changes in your management and riding styles. Be aware that traction devices can tear rubber mats, splinter wood flooring, and mar concrete and brick.

Any projection on a shoe presents an additional risk of serious injury from kicking when horses are turned out together. A horse is also at risk of cutting himself on traction devices when lying down.

Too much traction with certain kinds of footing can lead to sprains and strains. Always be aware of the type of terrain you are riding on and consider how much you are asking of your horse.

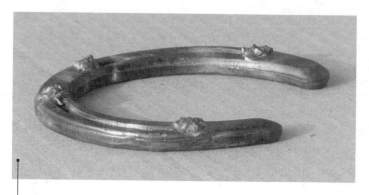

Borium

Traction materials with names like borium, Drill Tek, and EME can be applied to a horseshoe at the toe and/or heel in smears, beads, or points. These products generally consist of chips of very hard tungsten carbide in a softer carrier metal, typically bronze. Your farrier can use a forge or a heating torch to apply borium to a shoe. The bronze melts onto the shoe to hold the carbide chips in place. Borium greatly improves traction on very hard surfaces like concrete, ice, and rock and also increases the useful life of the shoes.

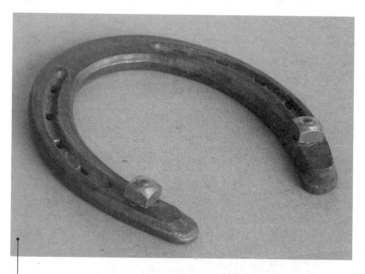

Studs

Calks or studs are projections of various sizes and configurations that are added to the ground surface of a shoe for added traction on soft or wet ground. Some are permanent and others, like the ones shown here, screw into threaded holes in the shoe and are removable.

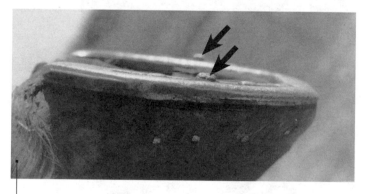

Ice Nails

Frost, mud, or ice nails that have tall, hardened heads can be substituted for regular horseshoe nails to provide added grip, especially on hard ground or ice. Often, two ice nails per shoe are all that are necessary to make a horse feel more confident on frozen ground. When ice nails are used at the midpoint of the hoof, as shown here, they can provide optimal traction without adversely affecting landing or breakover of the hoof. The regular nail heads in this shoe have worn down after four weeks, but the ice nails are still tall enough to provide added traction. (See also page 70.)

WINTER SHOEING

No matter what you use your horse for, if you ride outdoors in a temperate climate in the winter, your horse will require special hoof care.

When you are designing your winter hoof-care program, consider the natural conformation of your horse's hooves, the level and type of his winter exercise, the footing in exercise and turnout areas, the typical weather patterns in your locale, and the expertise of your farrier. Once you've considered all these factors, you might decide to have your horse's shoes pulled for the winter and ride him barefoot or with boots. Or you could have him shod with snow pads and borium or studs so he can train in all types of footing.

A barefoot horse with a naturally balanced hoof, a dense hoof horn, and a well-cupped sole is often able to grip many winter surfaces without hoof damage. And a naturally concave sole sheds snow, mud, and slush fairly well. However, a hoof with a long toe and low heel, brittle or punky horn, or a flat sole has poor traction, and the sole is vulnerable to bruising from frozen ground. Keep in mind that during the winter hooves have about half the rate of growth they have during the summer and therefore cannot stand a great deal of abrasive wear. Hoof boots can protect bare hooves during training and riding sessions and prevent snowballing. Some boots can be fitted with studs for more traction.

Many riders prefer to keep their horses shod for active winter riding. Shoes offer continuous hoof protection and maintain hoof balance. Winter shoes also can provide additional traction and prevent snowballing.

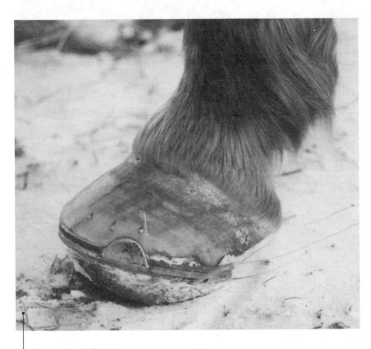

Snowballing

When mixtures of snow, ice, mud, manure, grass, or bedding accumulate in the sole area, it packs into dense ice mounds. These balls can seriously fatigue a horse's muscles, tendons, and joints as he constantly makes adjustments to keep his balance. It is easy for a snowballed horse to wrench a fetlock.

Applying various substances such as grease, petroleum jelly, silicone spray, or cooking spray to the sole of the hoof prevents snow buildup during certain temperatures but usually only for a few strides.

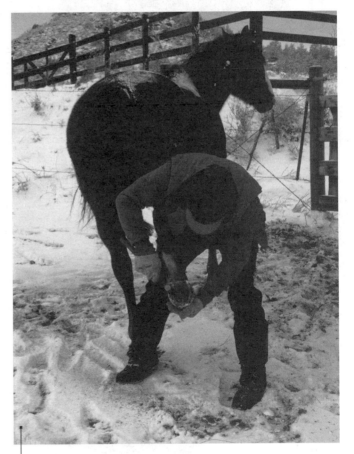

Depending on the snow's consistency and the temperature, snowballs can turn into dense ice balls and be almost impossible to chip out. A shod hoof is more prone to snowballing than a bare hoof because the junction of the inner edge of the shoe with the sole provides the perfect place for mud and ice to freeze and become securely lodged.

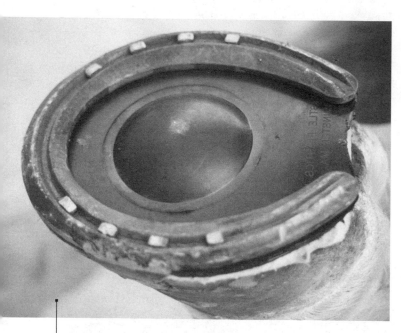

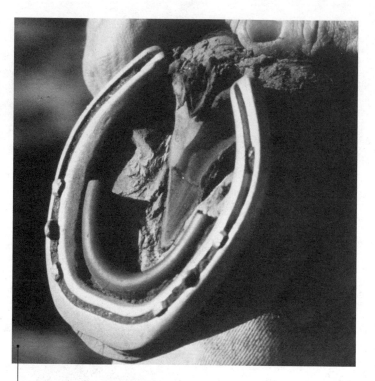

Bubble Pads Help Some

Full pads can help prevent snowballing in some situations, but they reduce traction because the natural cupped sole is covered. Full plastic pads with a convex bubble in the middle are only somewhat better than full flat pads at preventing snow buildup, but they provide even less traction because the bubble is often level with the shoe, preventing it from digging in.

Tube Pads Work Well

Tube-type rim pads that fit between the shoe and the hoof wall, leaving the sole open, are the best antisnow-balling option. The sole retains its cupped traction feature and can respire normally. As the horse's weight descends on the hoof, the tubes flex and dislodge the snow that accumulates at the junction of the shoe and the sole.

Cherry says . . .

TRY TUBES AND SMEARS FOR SNOW

When we're expecting our first snow, I ask Richard to put tube-type rim pads on all my shod horses. That way, whether they're lounging in their pen or pasture or I'm riding, they'll have minimal snowballing. If I plan to do a lot of road riding, I'll ask Richard to add a few borium smears to each shoe. That way, when we hit an icy spot, we'll have better traction.

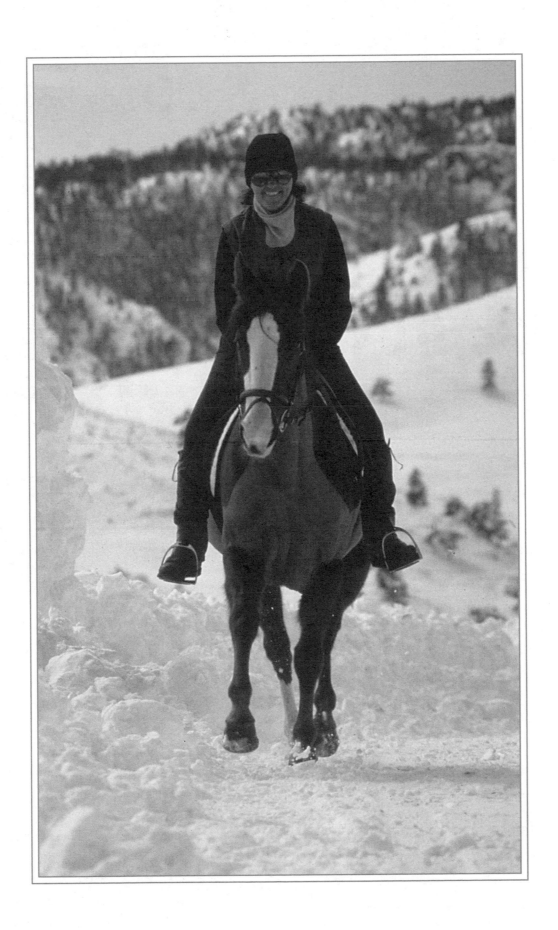

—9—
SHOEING,
AND HOW

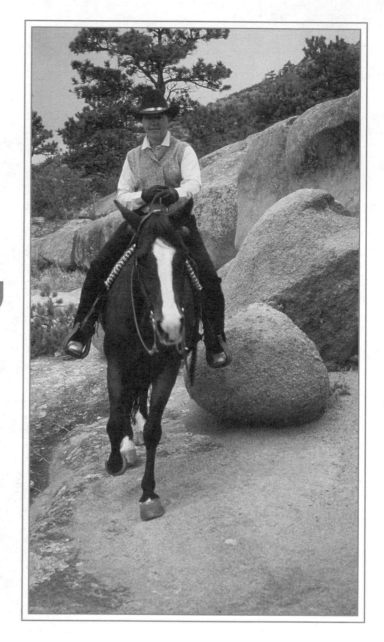

All farriers are blacksmiths, but not all blacksmiths are farriers. A blacksmith forges items from steel. A farrier shoes horses. Today, most blacksmiths do not shoe horses, and thus they are not farriers. Most farriers forge items from steel, so they are also blacksmiths.

A farrier can make, shape, and apply shoes hot or cold. Hot shoeing often refers to the use of a hammer and forge to make shoes from scratch or to modify keg shoes. Cold shoeing means the farrier shapes and applies the shoes without heating them. Many farriers use both hot- and cold-shoeing techniques.

Richard says . . .

COLD IS THE NORM

One of the nice things about using a forge to heat shoes is that is helps keep you warm in the winter. But, truth be told, the vast majority of my shoeing is done cold, without heating the shoes to shape them or to fit them to the hooves. I only hot-shoe when making and applying therapeutic shoes or specialty shoes like sliding plates or large draft horseshoes.

Like many farriers, I've found cold shoeing to be much more efficient for standard shoes. By using a stall jack, which is like a portable anvil on a stand, to shape the shoes cold, I can work close to the horse without having to travel back and forth to the forge in my truck. And not having to pull my truck into some barns and use a forge reduces the risk of fire in the barn.

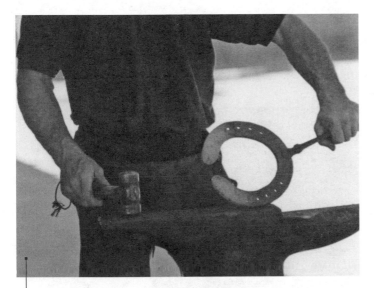

Hot Shaping
Large horseshoes must be heated in a forge to make the steel malleable for shaping.

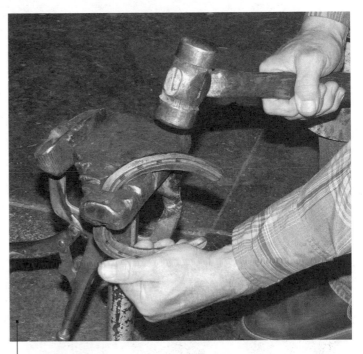

Cold Shaping
Most riding horseshoes can be shaped to fit the hoof without heating them.

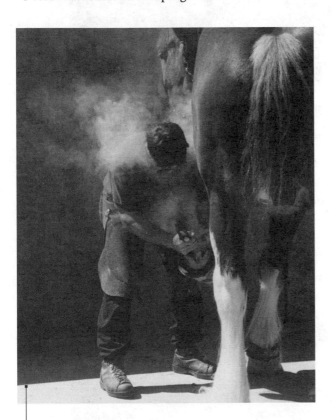

Hot Fitting
Hot fitting involves lightly touching a heated shoe to a hoof to mark "high spots" that need to be rasped for a perfect match. A final hot fit melts and seals the bottom of the hoof wall against invasion by environmental moisture. This does not hurt the horse, but the sound and smoke might startle him the first time.

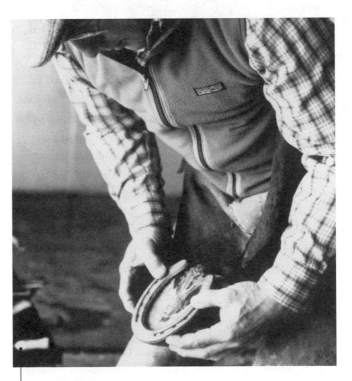

Cold Fitting
When cold fitting, a farrier needs to make sure both the shoe and the hoof are flat and level. Then the shoe will set solidly on the hoof without rocking, and there will be no gaps between them.

SHOEING STEPS

Each farrier develops his own shoeing methods and procedures, but the underlying principles remain the same: trim the hoof, fit the shoe to the hoof, nail the shoe on. By describing one shoeing process, we don't suggest that it is the only or the best way, but it should give you a better understanding of the many steps involved. Keep in mind that a barefoot trim will be different than a trim for shoeing (see page 50).

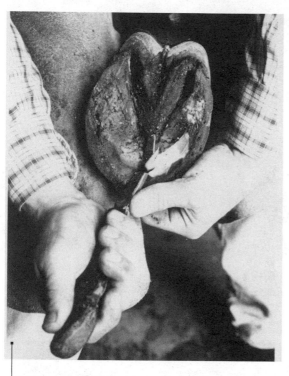

Trim the Sole
Evaluating and trimming the sole are the foundations of hoof balance. One of the most challenging and important things a farrier must learn, through training and experience, is how much sole to remove. Trimming a sole too thin can make a horse tender-footed and even lame. Leaving a sole too thick will not allow the hoof wall at the toe to be trimmed sufficiently to balance the hoof. This can result in low heels. A sole that's too thick also inhibits the natural expansion and springing action of the hoof capsule, an important shock-absorbing function of the hoof. The bars are trimmed only to remove overgrown, deformed horn.

Nip the Wall
The wall at the toe is trimmed to a level slightly longer than that of the sole. The heels are trimmed only enough to balance the hoof and to provide a strong base of support.

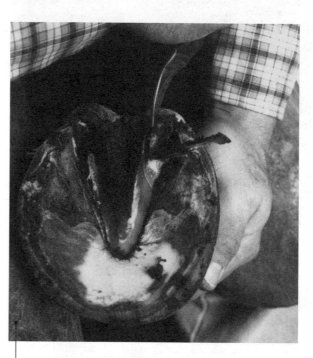

Trim the Frog
The frog is trimmed to remove loose and overgrown flaps that could trap dirt and manure and harbor anaerobic thrush organisms. The overgrown clefts of the frog at the heels should be trimmed so that the hoof can self-clean. This means that mud, manure, and other debris can exit the clefts at the rear of the hoof. The frog provides traction and secondary support in soft footing, but it is not necessary for the frog to bear weight when the horse is standing on hard, level ground.

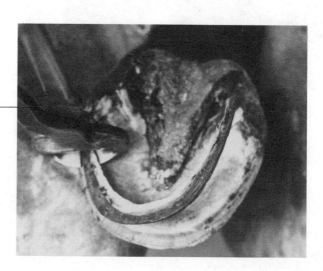

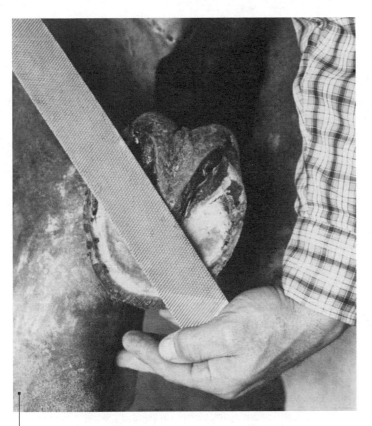

Rasp the Hoof

The bottom of the hoof is rasped flat and level.

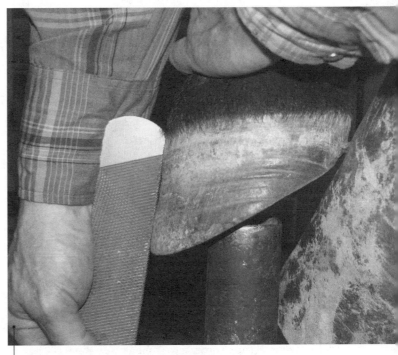

Check for Flares and Dishes

The hoof wall is checked for flares at the quarters and for a dish at the toe. These dips or curves weaken the hoof. A straight edge, such as that of a rasp, held against the hoof wall can help identify flares and dishes.

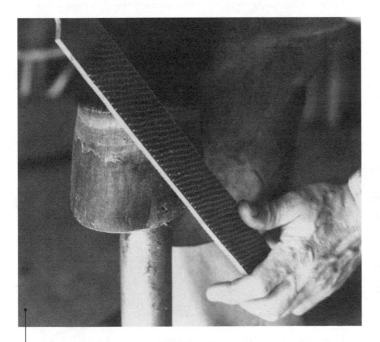

Dressing Flares from the Top

A hoof should be dressed (rasped) to remove flares and dishes every time the hoof is trimmed to ensure that the hoof wall is true from the coronet to the ground.

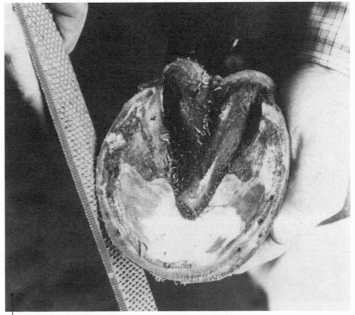

Dressing Flares from the Bottom

The farrier can also remove a flare and shape the hoof from the bottom by pulling the rasp toward him.

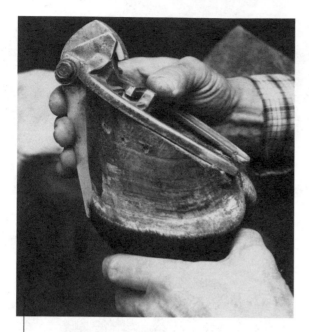

Measure the Hoof Angle

A hoof gauge (hoof protractor) measures the angle between the hoof wall at the toe and the bottom of the hoof, which corresponds to the angle between the front of the hoof and the ground when the horse is standing on a flat, level surface.

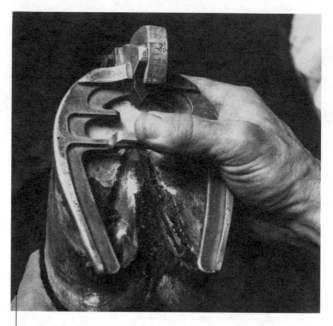

Read the Hoof Angle

Recording a horse's ideal hoof angles after a balanced trim can help ensure that the horse is trimmed the same way each time, whether by the same farrier or a different one. Some farriers, however, prefer to rely solely on their eyes when balancing a hoof. What is really important is the angle of the coffin bone in relation to the ground (see page 3).

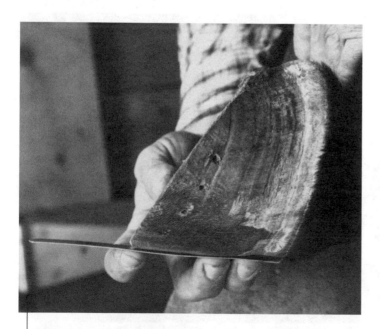

Measure the Toe Length

Using calipers or a special hoof ruler as shown here, toe length is measured from the soft indentation at the top of the hoof (the coronary band) to the ground surface.

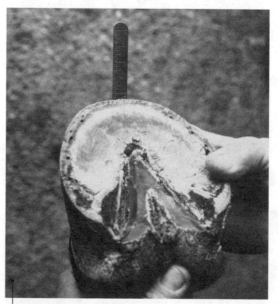

Compare Toe Measurements

Toe-length measurements can help a farrier trim pairs of hooves to match. They also can help ensure that the hooves are trimmed to the same length each time, whether the same farrier or a different one does it.

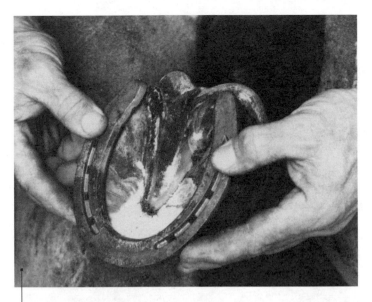

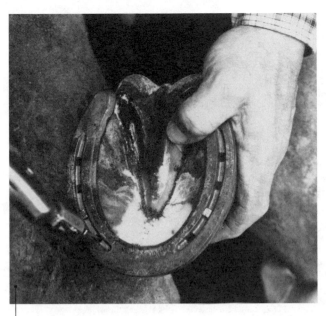

Fit the Shoe

Once the shoe is shaped, the farrier holds it on the hoof to check the fit and to make sure that it sets flat against the hoof.

Nail the Shoe

Holding the shoe in position on the hoof with one hand, the farrier drives one nail to secure the shoe.

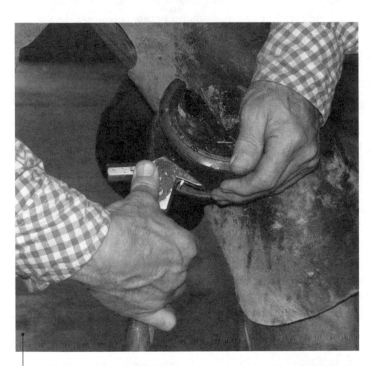

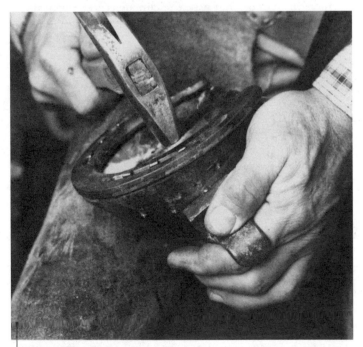

Twist Off the Nail Ends

As each nail is driven, the farrier uses the claw of the hammer to twist the end of the nail off so he won't be injured if the horse jerks his leg. The remaining stub will form the clinch. He then drives the remaining nails, usually a total of six. When applying a keg shoe, heel nails are usually not used, to avoid restricting normal expansion of the hoof.

Block the Clinches

Holding a hardened steel block under each clinch, the farrier strikes the head of each nail in turn with a hammer. This sets the clinch, bending it sharply where it exits the hoof wall so it pulls the shoe firmly against the hoof. This also seats the head of the nail firmly in the crease of the shoe.

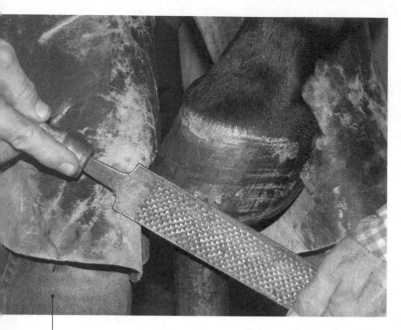

File Under the Clinches

The farrier files all the clinches to a uniform length. He uses the edge of the rasp to smooth the hoof wall where the nails exited. That way, the clinches can be bent flat against the hoof.

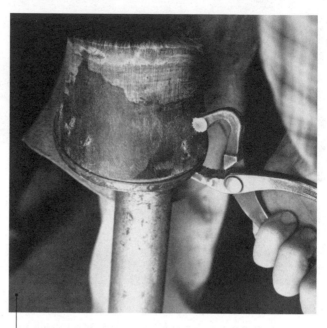

Close the Clinches

A clincher is used to bend the clinches down and set them flat against the hoof wall. The curved jaw of the clincher presses on and bends the clinch, while the opposing straight jaw pushes against the nail head to keep it seated.

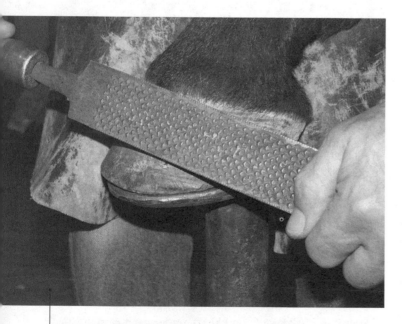

File the Clinches Smooth

The clinches are filed smooth and flush with the hoof wall to prevent the horse from cutting his face if he rubs against his hoof or from cutting the hands of a person handling the hoof.

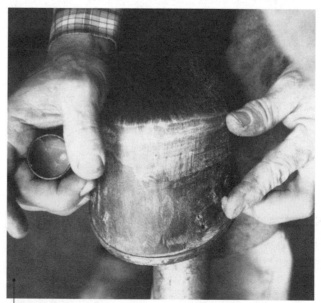

Fill the Holes

Nail holes, old and new, are filled with wax to keep dirt and moisture from entering the hoof. If the hoof wall was rasped extensively to remove flares, a hoof sealer is applied and allowed to dry before the nail holes are filled with wax.

THE HORSESHOE NAIL

When a horseshoe nail is driven into the hoof properly, it will neither cause the horse pain nor injure the hoof. But an improperly driven nail can do both.

The nail should be driven through the thickest part of the hoof wall; this is insensitive tissue similar in consistency to wood. Tissues beneath the hoof wall are rich in blood and nerve vessels, and driving a nail into these tissues can cause intense pain and profuse bleeding. The white line is the dividing line between sensitive and insensitive layers and is used as a guideline for driving nails.

Nail Paths

A driven nail is good, close, or hot.

A good nail **(A)** enters the hoof somewhere within the boundaries of the white line and curves outward to exit the hoof wall at a point about one-third the distance from the hoof bottom to the coronary band.

A close nail **(B)** puts pressure on sensitive inner tissues (also known as "the quick") without actually piercing them. A close nail might cause the horse immediate discomfort or could go unnoticed for many days or until the horse is put into work. Usually it can be located by the use of a hoof tester or by light tapping with a hammer at each clinch. Removal of the close nail will often return the horse to soundness with no further attention needed, since sensitive structures have not been invaded.

A hot nail **(C)** is one that has been driven into sensitive tissue — "quicking" a horse. It will usually cause an immediate pain reaction, and the horse will pull his foot away, unless he is under sedation for shoeing. If a horse is normally fractious and is constantly jerking his foot when being shod, the response to a hot nail might not be noticed. When a hot nail is removed, blood will likely be seen in the nail hole and on the nail. The hole will need to be flushed by your farrier or veterinarian with an antiseptic such as Betadine and packed to prevent contamination. A nail should not be used in that hole of the shoe. The horse should be current on his tetanus vaccination and should be observed for several days for developing lameness.

If lameness does develop, the hoof is likely infected, and a veterinarian should be contacted. A common treatment requires shoe removal and soaking the hoof in a solution of hot water and Epsom salt twice daily for two to three days using a hoof-soaking boot or a bucket. Between soakings, a hoof boot or bandages will protect the hoof and keep it clean. When the veterinarian determines that the infection has cleared, the shoe can be replaced.

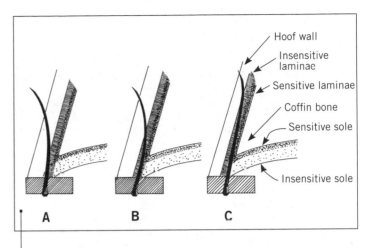

Nail Paths
A. A good nail   B. A close nail   C. A hot nail

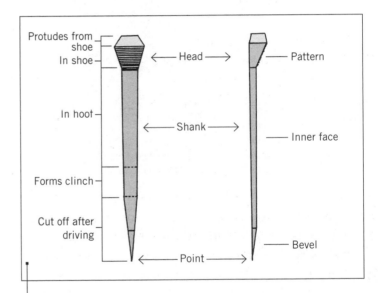

Parts of a Nail

The point of every horseshoe nail is beveled on one side, and the shank of the nail curves away from the bevel when it is driven into the hoof wall. The head of the nail has a pattern on the same side as the bevel so the farrier can tell by sight and by feel how to position the nail for driving. The pattern on the head is always positioned toward the center of the hoof. Most of the nail head seats into the crease in the shoe, where it is protected from wearing off. The very top of the head, about 1/16 inch (0.16 cm), protrudes from the shoe.

NEW SHOES OR RESET?

Generally, if the branches of the shoe are wearing evenly, horseshoes can be reset until the crease is no longer deep enough to protect the nail heads. If optimal traction is critical for a performance, new shoes may be required at each shoeing.

Shoe wear is affected by the type of shoe; the kind and amount of riding and exercise the horse gets; and the footing he trains, works, and lives on. Some horses wear out a set of steel shoes in five weeks, with very little riding time; others might have their shoes reset two or more times before new shoes are required. The decision of whether to reset or replace shoes is best left to your farrier.

More often than not, a shoe will have to be reshaped, however slightly, before it is reset onto the trimmed hoof. Many farriers charge the same fee for a reset as they do for new shoes because it takes the same or more time to clean and reshape the shoes for reset as it does to prepare new shoes.

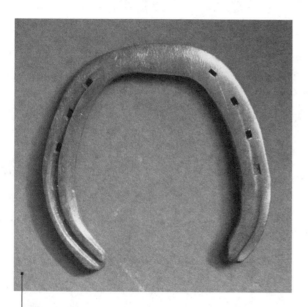

Shoe Wear on the Ground Surface

When a shoe like the rim shoe shown in this photo is worn too thin to protect the nail heads or to give sufficient support to the foot, it is time to replace it. Normal wear that a shoe receives at the toe rounds the front edge of the shoe so it resembles a new rolled-toe shoe (see page 63). This shape is often beneficial to a horse's movement and is one advantage to resetting shoes.

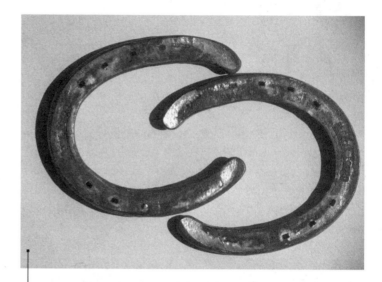

Shoe Wear on the Hoof Surface

Each time the horse takes a step, the heels of the hoof expand and contract, moving imperceptibly on the shoe. Evidence of this repetitive heel movement can be seen as a shiny strip of polished steel on most shoes when they are removed. But sometimes, as with the pair of front shoes shown here, these grooves are worn so deeply that there is no longer a flat shoe surface to provide sufficient support for the hoof, and new shoes for the horse are necessary.

Cherry says . . .

SAME OLD SHOES

After being married to a farrier for so many years, I have to chuckle when I hear other horse owners complain that their farrier sometimes reuses the same shoes instead of putting on new shoes every time. Blame it on my upbringing, but it has always seemed wasteful to me to throw something out that is still perfectly useful, horseshoes included.

–10–
OWNER
SKILLS

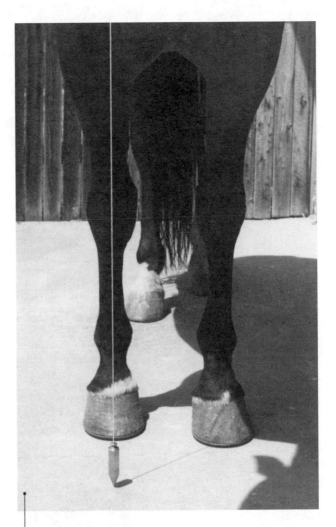

Side-to-Side Balance
Medial-lateral (ML) balance is the anatomical way of describing the balance between the inside (medial) wall of the hoof and the outside (lateral) wall of the hoof. As you look at the horse from the front, the hoof should be centered under the leg. This will allow the hoof to bear weight evenly. A plumb bob or weight on a string will help you train your eye.

As a horse owner, learning how to handle your horse safely and effectively and training him to be mannerly will help your farrier and veterinarian do their best work when your horse needs them. Also, developing your eye so you can tell what is normal with your horse's behavior, stance, movement, and appearance can help you determine when something is amiss that might require the attention of a professional.

KNOW GOOD WORK
WHEN YOU SEE IT

One very important skill is being able to recognize a good shoeing job when you see it. Shoeing affects your horse's immediate performance and his long-term soundness. You might not think you need to pay much attention to your horse's shoeing as long as your horse is not lame and his shoes stay on. While it's true that horses are very adaptable and resilient and can often tolerate poor shoeing for months or even years, it's possible that by the time signs of lameness appear, your horse's hooves might be irreparably damaged. Shoeing methods aimed at keeping shoes on as the number-one priority often bypass other important shoeing principles and could put your horse out of commission for good.

There are many guidelines for judging shoeing quality, some of which are more important than others. You can easily evaluate the basic aspects of a farrier's work with a pencil and a flat, level surface for your horse to stand on. Try to make the evaluation within the first week or two of shoeing because hooves can quickly change shape as they grow.

Keep in mind that these tips are general guidelines for assessing your horse's shoeing. Every hoof must be shod individually, taking into consideration the horse's conformation, movement, habits, management, and intended use.

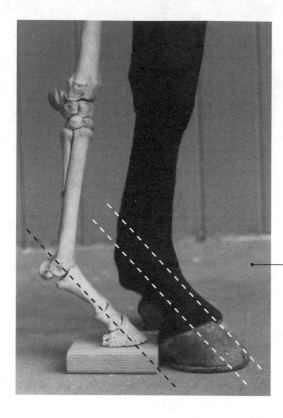

Hoof and Pastern Angles

Dorsal-palmar (DP) balance is the anatomical way of describing how the hoof angle lines up with the pastern angle. DP balance is generally correct when, viewed from the side, the front (dorsal) surface of the hoof is parallel to an imaginary line passing through the center of the pastern.

Checking DP Balance

With the horse standing square (cannons perpendicular to the ground) move 8 to 10 feet (2.4–3 m) from the side of the horse and crouch down to view the feet. Hold a pencil at arm's length and line it up with the center axis of a pastern. The front of the hoof should be parallel with the pencil.

If the hoof angle is too low, the junction where the lines of the hoof and pastern meet will be "broken back." If the hoof angle is too high, the imaginary line will be "broken forward" (see page 3). Of the two, a broken-back axis is more common, and more harmful, as it is associated with long-toe/low-heel syndrome.

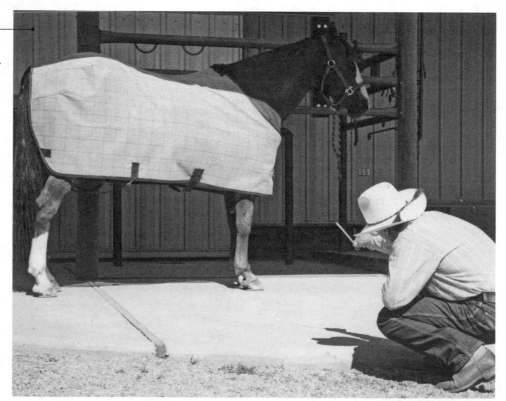

Heel Support

A shoe should extend beyond the heels of a hoof so that the limb is adequately supported. Generally the heel of a shoe should be below the midline of the cannon bone when the cannon is vertical. Short shoeing — using a horseshoe that is too short for the hoof — is one of the most common and potentially harmful shoeing errors. Shoes that are too short will not provide adequate support for the limb and can result in underrun heels, fatigue, and permanent damage to the horse's limbs (see below).

Because horses commonly lose front shoes when their hind hooves step on and pull off the exposed heels of the front shoes, many horseshoers are hesitant to extend the heels of the shoe. They figure it will save them a return trip to replace a lost shoe. Horses with well-formed upright hooves are better able to tolerate short shoeing without permanent damage than are horses with lower angles or underrun heels.

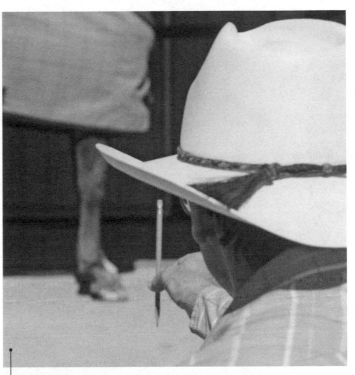

Check Heel Length

To check heel length, while still crouched 8 to 10 feet (2.4–3 m) away from the horse, hold the pencil at arm's length and line it up with an imaginary line that runs through the center of the cannon bone to the ground. Generally, the heels of the shoe should reach this line or extend behind it. The more the heels are underrun, the farther the shoe needs to extend behind the hoof in order to provide necessary support. In many cases, egg bar shoes or shoes with long extended heels that don't join (sometimes called "open egg bars") are used to provide support for underrun heels.

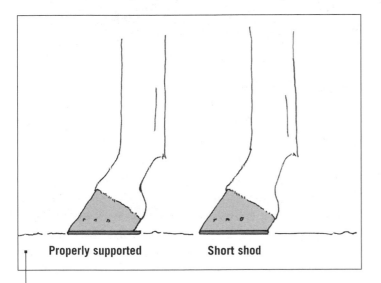

Properly supported   **Short shod**

Short Shoeing

Applying shoes that are too small is called "short shoeing." The shoes are fit tight to the foot with no extra shoe at the quarters for expansion or extending past the heels for support. Short shoeing is done out of fear that a horse will step on an exposed heel and pull the shoe off, although this is unlikely to happen if the feet are properly balanced.

While a horse can usually survive one or two cycles of short shoeing with no permanent damage, over the long term it will likely end up costing more in soundness than your horse has in his health savings account.

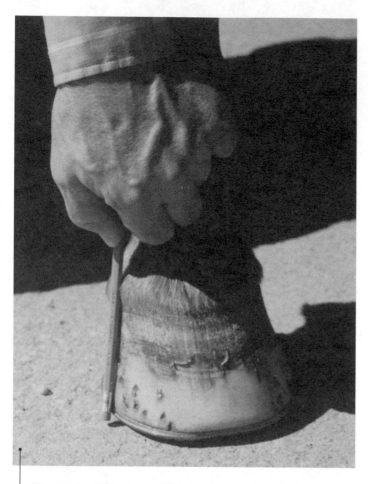

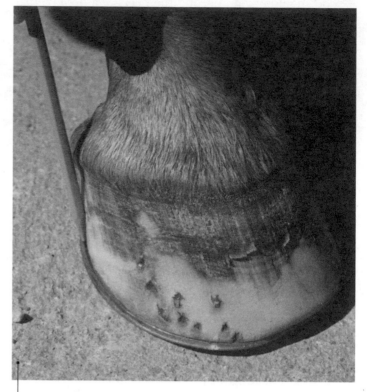

Check for Flares and Dishes

A **flare** is a concave bend, or dip, in the hoof. A flare at the toe is called a **dish**. A hoof is strongest when the hoof wall running the entire length of the hoof — from the coronary band to the ground — is true, without flares or dishes. Most hooves tend to develop flares and dishes to some degree, but they can usually be kept in check if a shoer takes the time to "dress" the hoof wall true with a rasp every time the horse is trimmed.

To check if a hoof is developing a flare or a dish, lay a pencil against the hoof wall, starting just below the coronet and extending past the bottom of the hoof. A space under the center of the pencil indicates a flare or a dish. Whether or not flares are kept under control by careful shaping of the hoof often makes the difference between a good shoer and a fast shoer.

Check Expansion

Expansion is the amount of shoe that extends past the sides of the hoof at the heels. Although the shoe should fit flush with the hoof from the toe around to the quarters (the widest part of the foot) when the horse is freshly shod, the shoe needs to be wider than the hoof from the quarters to the heels by at least the thickness of a dime. That is because the hoof is cone shaped and it gets larger (i.e., expands) at the bottom as it grows longer. Also, the hoof expands (gets wider) across the heels every time the horse puts weight on the foot (see page 80, photo on right). A metal horseshoe does not change size or shape once it is applied to a hoof, so to provide room for normal growth and hoof movement, a shoe needs to be made large enough to accommodate the hoof not only on the day of shoeing, but six weeks down the road. By that time, the hoof has grown wider and is flush with the edge of the shoe.

You can check for expansion by running the blunt point of a pencil around the edge of the shoe from the quarter back to the heel. If there's no shoe edge for the pencil to ride on, there's no expansion room. Note: A squared toe shoe or a shoe intentionally set back by the farrier will not fit flush with the hoof at the toe.

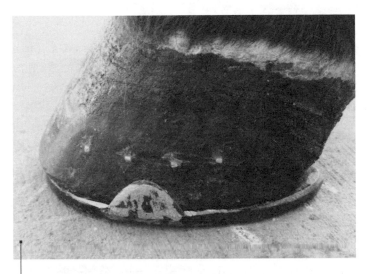

Nail Pattern and Clinches

The nail pattern is affected by the quality of the hoof, the skill of the farrier, and the quality and design of the shoes and nails being used. The height of the nail farthest back on the shoe should be approximately one-third the distance up from the ground to the coronary band. Ideally, the nail pattern should form a straight line that is level or sloped slightly downward toward the toe. The two toe nails should be the same height when viewed from the front of the hoof.

The clinches should be uniform in size, and the visible part should look square, with all sides equal. Clinches should set flush with the hoof wall. A groove should not be filed in the hoof wall as a place to recess the clinches because the groove would weaken the hoof.

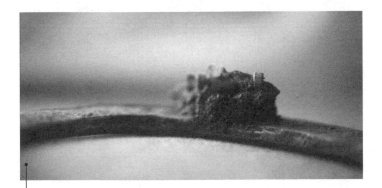

Large Clinches Can Damage the Hoof

Large rectangular clinches that are longer than they are wide can really hold a shoe on, but they can also cause problems. If the shoe is stepped on or caught on something and pulled off, large clinches will usually rip off large portions of the hoof, requiring extra work for your farrier to repair and more expense for you.

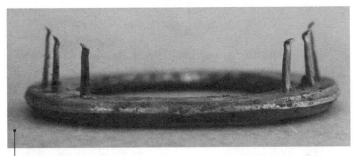

Clinches Should Open if the Shoe Gets Caught

Square clinches will hold the shoe securely yet open easily to allow the shoe to come off without damaging the hoof if the shoe gets caught on something.

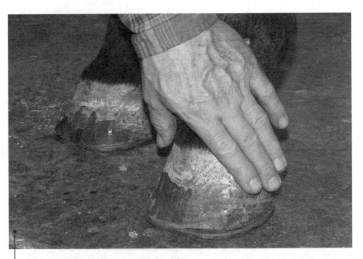

Smooth Clinches

Clinches should be smooth when you run your hand over them. If your hands aren't as tough as the farrier's in this photo, you might want to use a cloth or wear a cotton glove so you don't cut your hand if there's a metal burr.

ASK QUESTIONS

As the owner, you are ultimately responsible for providing your horse with proper hoof care. If his shoeing varies significantly from these guidelines, or if you have questions about the way he is shod, talk with your farrier. A good shoer will not be offended by straightforward questions and should be able to explain in terms you can understand why he's shoeing your horse in a particular manner. If he is unwilling or unable to provide satisfactory answers, it might be time to think about putting your horse's feet in the hands of another farrier.

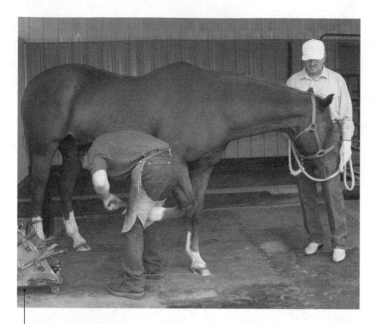

Out in the Open
When holding the horse out in the open, stand on the opposite side of the horse from the farrier so you can keep the horse in position if he starts to move away from the farrier.

HOLDING A HORSE FOR THE FARRIER

There may be times when you'll need to hold a horse for the farrier because there is no safe place to tie him for shoeing or because the horse is better behaved when he's held. How effectively you hold and handle a horse for shoeing can make a big difference in his behavior and, consequently, the quality of the farrier's job. It's easy to daydream or become distracted, but if you focus on your job, it will enable the farrier to do his.

When holding the horse, keep his head straight and still to help him maintain steady balance on three legs. Don't let him nuzzle or slobber on the farrier. Horses can move suddenly and with great force, and a farrier can be seriously injured if the handler is not paying attention.

Where to Stand

Where you stand when holding your horse for the farrier will depend on your facilities, your horse, and your farrier's preference.

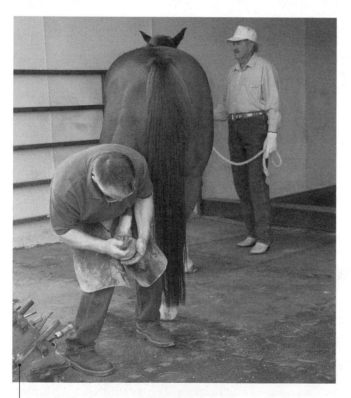

Control the Horse's Head
When the farrier is working on a hind, keep the horse's head forward and his body straight. If you let the horse turn his neck around to see what's going on, it can make the farrier's job harder as he supports the shifting weight of the horse.

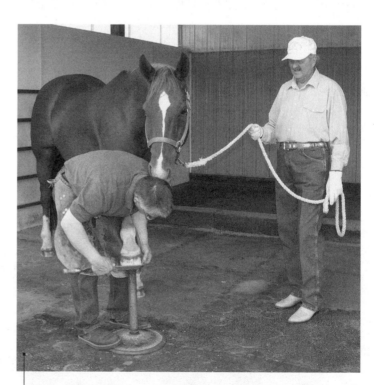

Watch Your Horse, Not the Farrier's Hands!
Standing on the opposite side of the horse from the farrier will give the farrier room to work when he brings the front leg forward. Although it is natural for a horse to inspect something in his blind spot, watch your horse and keep him from biting, nibbling, nuzzling, or slobbering on the farrier!

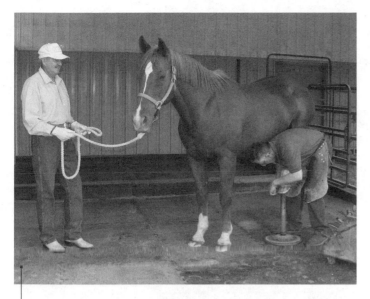

Let the Horse Find His Balance

When the farrier brings the horse's hind leg forward to set it on his knee or on the hoof stand, give the horse enough lead rope so he can lower his head a bit if he needs to. A lower head will help some horses balance in this position.

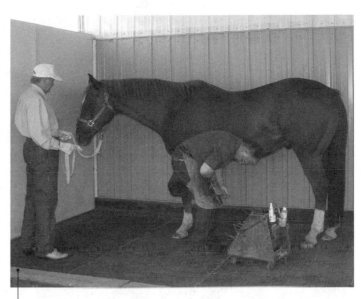

Against a Wall

When holding the horse along a wall or rail, stand on the same side as the farrier. The wall will keep the horse from moving away from the farrier.

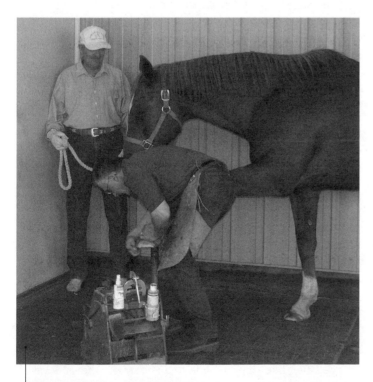

Don't Get Trapped in a Corner

When the farrier brings the front leg forward, you'll need to give him room to work. But don't box yourself into a corner as shown here. If the horse should rear or slip off the hoof stand, you could be injured.

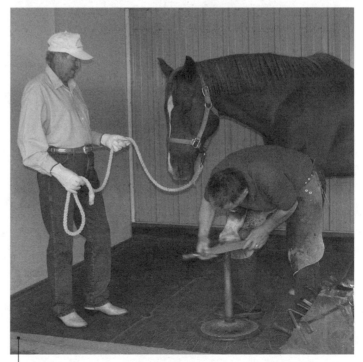

Leave Room to Maneuver

To keep from being boxed in, move the horse away from the wall so you have space to maneuver if the horse acts up or if his foot slips off the hoof stand.

REMOVING A SHOE

There will likely come a time when you'll need to remove a shoe that has bent or has shifted on the hoof and is unsafe. Practice before that day arrives, preferably under the guidance of your farrier, so when the time comes you will be able to remove the shoe successfully without injuring yourself or your horse.

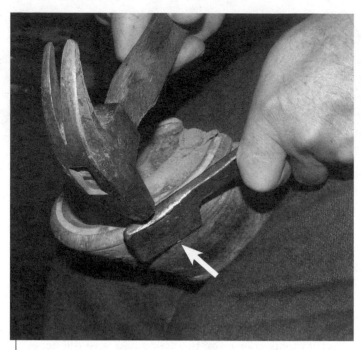

Finding the Clinches Can Be a Challenge

With practice, you may be able to position the clinch cutter by feel. Otherwise, you will need to bend way over to see where the clinches are.

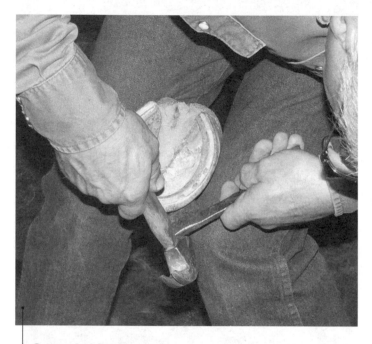

Open the Clinches

To remove a shoe, first open the clinches so that the nails can slide through the hoof wall when you pull the shoe. Holding the foot between your knees, place the sharp edge of the clinch cutter against the end of one clinch and then strike the opposite edge of the clinch cutter with a hammer to drive the cutter under the clinch and bend it open. Repeat the maneuver until all of the clinches are open.

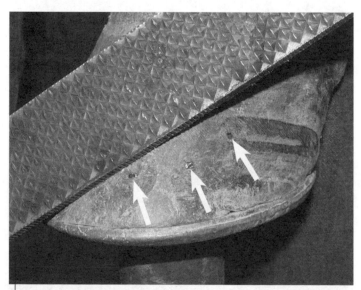

Filing Off the Clinches

An alternative to using a clinch cutter and hammer is to use a file, like the fine side of a shoeing rasp, to file off the clinches. This is made easier by placing the hoof on a hoof stand. A drawback to this method is that inexperienced hands will abrade much of the protective outer hoof layer and you could end up with damaging furrows in the hoof wall where each clinch used to be.

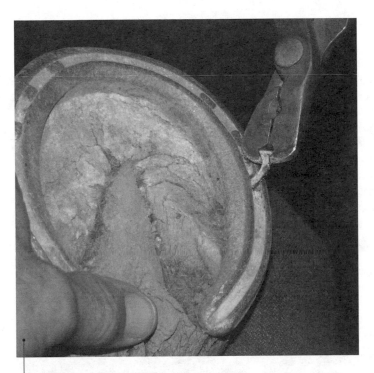

Pull Each Nail Individually

The least stressful way to remove the shoe once the clinches have been opened or filed off is to use a crease nail puller. Grab the head of each nail, and pry out one by one. The first pry will get a nail partway out, then loosen your grip and grab the nail shank closer to the shoe to complete the extraction.

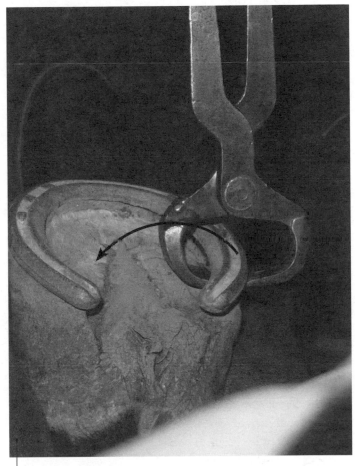

Using Pull-Offs

As an alternative to pulling the nails individually, you can use pull-offs to pry the shoe and nails from the hoof after opening or filing the clinches. Begin by working the jaws of the pull-offs under one heel of the shoe and prying toward the center of the frog.

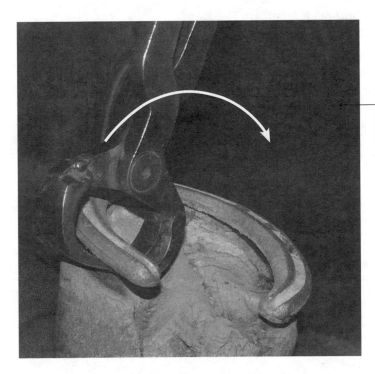

Pry the Other Heel

Do the same with the other heel. Just loosen the shoe at this point — don't be in a hurry.

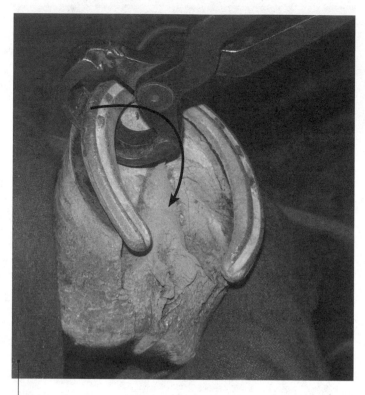

Work Your Way around the Shoe . . .

Work your way toward the toe, always prying toward the center of the hoof. If you pry toward the outside, you risk breaking the hoof wall.

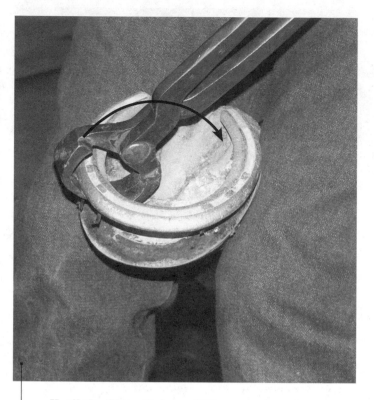

. . . Until the Shoe Comes Off

Pry the shoe from the other side. By now, the shoe may be loose enough to come off. If not, go around again, prying the heels and then the sides.

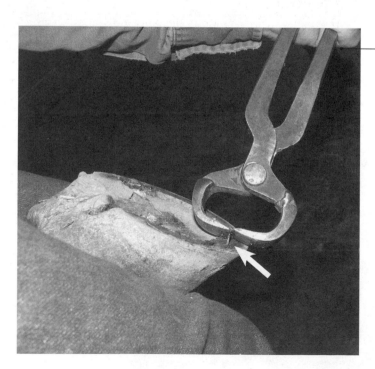

Remove Nails from the Hoof

Once the shoe is off, check that no nails remain in the hoof. Sometimes the nails break off or heads are worn so small that they slide through the holes in a shoe and stay in the hoof. If you spot a vagrant nail, grab it with the pull-offs and pry it out of the hoof.

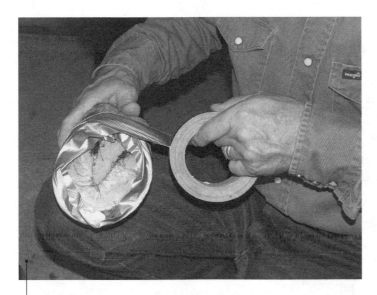

Protect the Hoof with Tape

If your horse has tough hooves and you have a soft, nonabrasive place (like a bedded stall) to keep him until the farrier can replace the shoe, you can likely leave the hoof bare. But in most cases it's good insurance to protect the edge of the hoof from chipping by wrapping it with duct tape, stretch wrap, or other material until the farrier arrives.

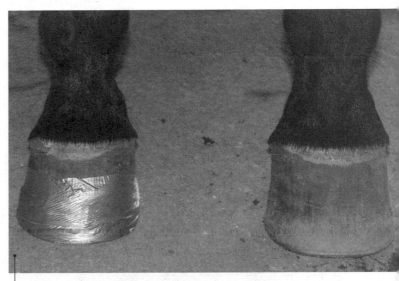

Check Protective Hoof Wrap for Wear

Tape and other hoof wrap wear away quickly if the ground is abrasive or the horse is very active. Check the wrap often to make sure the hoof is not being damaged.

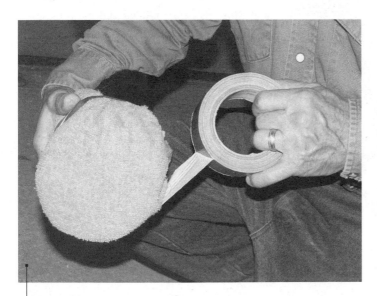

Protect a Sensitive Sole

If your horse is very sensitive walking on his sole without the shoe or if he will be in a rocky pen or on other footing that might bruise his sole, tape a towel or a hoof pad to the bottom of his hoof for temporary protection.

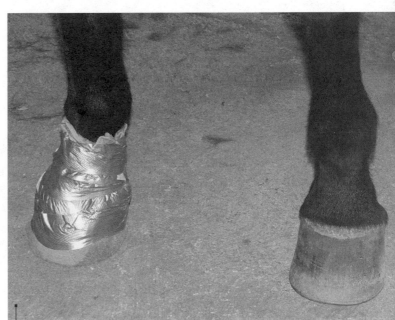

Practice Before a Shoe Is Lost

It's a good idea to accustom your horse to the sound of duct tape coming off the roll and to the feel of a towel around each of his feet long before you need to use that method. If you practice wrapping each of your horse's hooves, you'll have a much better chance of the process going smoothly when your horse does lose a shoe.

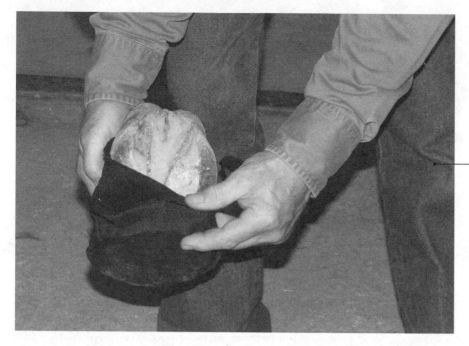

Emergency Boots

Using an emergency hoof boot is a quick and effective way to protect your horse's hoof from damage until the farrier arrives. As with a hoof wrap, practice applying a boot to each of your horse's feet so when an emergency arises you both will be comfortable with the process.

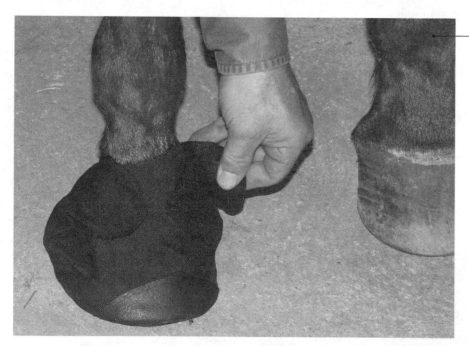

Have a Boot for Every Hoof

Be sure to have boots on hand that will fit your horse's front hooves and his hinds. Some boots, like the one shown here, are loose in form and will fit a wide range of sizes. With other more rigid boots you may need to have more than one size on hand.

APPLYING HOOF PRODUCTS

The hoof has two natural protective coverings, the periople and the stratum tectorum. Both layers retard moisture movement from the outside environment into the hoof and from the inside of the hoof to the outside. If the thin layer of stratum tectorum is rasped away, you should apply hoof sealer to replace it. However, because a healthy, strong hoof is naturally dry and hard, it is not usually a good practice to apply hoof dressing that softens the hoof. Avoid products containing petroleum or solvents like acetone and turpentine that can emulsify the hoof's natural oils and dry it out. Never apply grease or motor oil to the hooves. Used motor oil is especially bad because it contains toxins and carcinogens.

Cherry says . . .

APPLY WATER BEFORE HOOF DRESSING

When conditioning leather, I recommend applying the conditioner to slightly damp leather. As the leather dries, the oil is drawn into the leather. Our dermatologist recommends applying moisturizer to damp hands, feet, and face for the same reason. Therefore, when applying hoof dressing to cracked heel bulbs, use a brush and clean water to clean the area, and apply the dressing while the bulbs are still moist, or apply after a bath.

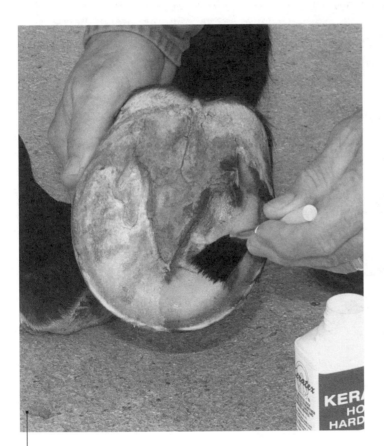

Hardener for the Sole

Hoof hardeners react chemically with the hoof to make it stronger and tougher. They can be useful for strengthening poor-quality hooves and thin, weak soles. Make sure the sole is clean and dry before applying the hardener. After you've applied it, hold the foot up for a minute or so to let the hardener soak in before setting it down.

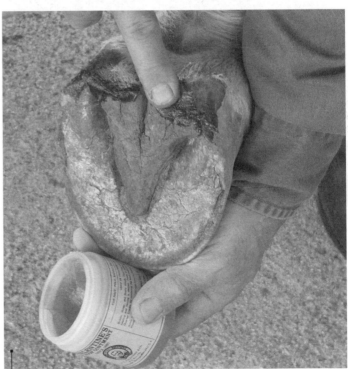

Hoof Dressing for Dry Heel Bulbs

One time hoof dressing is warranted is when the bulbs of the heels have become so dry that they are beginning to flake and crack. In order to restore pliability to the heel bulbs, rub a product that contains animal fat (such as lanolin or fish oil) into the heels daily until the desired result has been achieved. Before applying a hoof product, make sure that the hoof is clean.

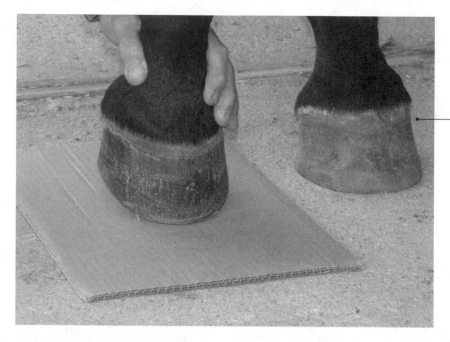

Use Cardboard to Protect the Floor

Before you bend down and open a bottle of hoof polish or sealer next to your horse's foot, train him to stand calmly while you place a piece of cardboard under his hoof. Practice placing the cardboard under each hoof until he's comfortable with the procedure, and he'll stand for several minutes without moving. When you apply hoof products, the cardboard will keep the applicator clean and prevent those telltale circular stains on the barn floor.

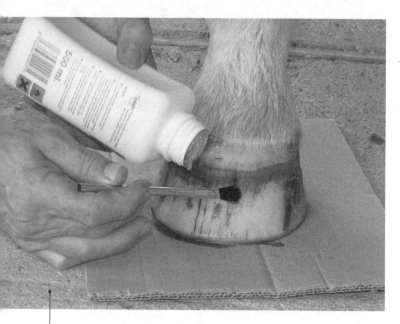

Hoof-Sealer Gel

Good hoof-sealer gels or liquids are semipermeable. They protect the hoof from the harmful effects of decomposing manure and urine. They also prevent excess water from entering the hoof, while still allowing moisture from normal hoof respiration to be released. Hoof sealers make the hoof less likely to soften and weaken in wet conditions. What you don't want to use is an airtight, waterproof barrier like varnish or shellac that will prevent normal hoof respiration. Apply gel hoof sealers to a clean, dry hoof.

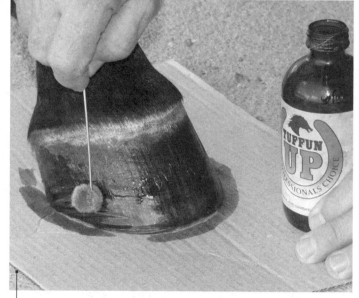

Hoof-Sealer Liquid

Be sure the hoof is clean and dry. Start applying a thin, even coat of liquid hoof sealer about ½ inch (1.3 cm) below the coronary band, and work your way down the hoof. Avoid the sensitive skin of the coronary band, which could become irritated. And there is no need to seal the periople that covers the hoof wall just below the coronet; the periople is already nature's best hoof sealer.

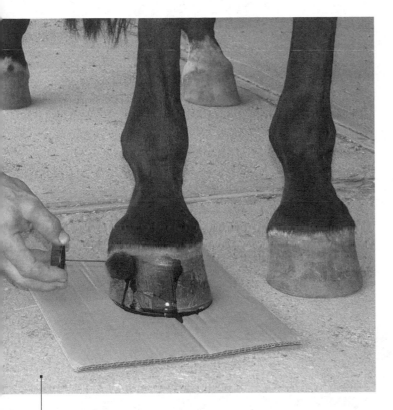

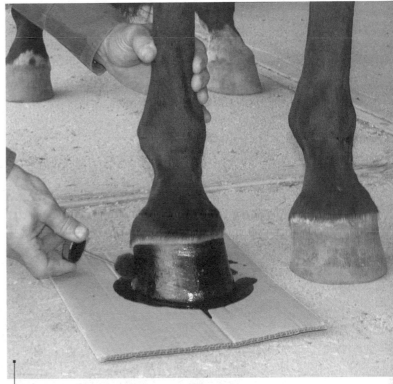

Hoof Polish

Hoof polish can be clear or black and is used to make the hooves look neat and shiny for horse shows. Make sure the hoof is clean and dry before applying hoof polish. Clip hair around the coronary band to make a tidy border, and be careful not to apply polish over the coronary band because it might irritate the skin. Start at the top, and apply hoof polish in overlapping horizontal lines until you reach the bottom.

Be careful, and keep your hand steady when applying hoof black to the top of the hoof because an uneven line will be more noticeable than with clear polish, especially on a foot with white hair.

Hold Steady until Polish Dries

To prevent dirt from sticking to the hoof, keep your horse on a clean, dry surface, such as concrete or a rubber mat, until the polish dries. When you've finished, stand back and walk all around your horse to check his hooves from all angles to see if you've missed any spots.

Cherry says . . .

NO CROOKED LINES

When showing in halter classes, the correctness and symmetry of your horse's limbs and hooves are being evaluated. So take extra care to do a neat job with hoof polish so the hooves don't look crooked, deformed, or asymmetrical.

HOOF POLISH TIPS

Prepare the hoof surface carefully. If the hoof has a rough or uneven surface, it can be smoothed with sandpaper before applying hoof shine. Start with coarse sandpaper, and work your way down to fine sandpaper and then, finally, to steel wool. The consequence of sanding the hoof is that it removes the natural protective stratum tectorum hoof layer. You might think that's okay because you will be applying hoof polish to replace it, but in fact, some hoof polish forms an airtight, waterproof barrier that can be harmful to the hoof if used for extended periods.

After a show, remove hoof polish and apply a quality hoof sealer or hoof hardener to protect the hoof. Water-based polish can be removed with soap and water, while others need polish remover, acetone, or another recommended solvent. Many solvents are drying to hooves.

Here are some other tips:

- To minimize the harmful effects of hoof polish, first apply a good-quality sealer or hardener, let it dry, and then apply the polish.
- To repel dust and keep the polish looking shiny and "wet," apply polish enhancer over the polish.
- Place the bottle of polish in a tin can so if hoof black drips down the side of the bottle it won't get on your hands or make a ring where you set it down.
- Pour a small amount into an extra bottle so if the bottle tips over you won't spill as much and you'll still have some to finish the job.
- Apply a dab of petroleum jelly or cooking spray on the threads of the bottle to prevent the cap from getting glued shut.

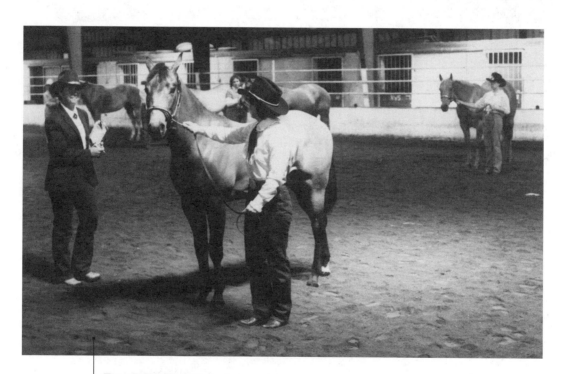

Read the Rules

If you plan on showing your horse, it's up to you to become familiar with the show regulations regarding shoeing and hoof polish. Some shows have specific rules regarding size and weight of shoes and use of pads. Others, like the Foundation Quarter Horse Association or Appaloosa Horse Club, prohibit the use of hoof black in all or certain classes. You can get show guidelines online or from the show organization (see Resource Guide).

-11-
HOOF PROBLEMS AND FIXES

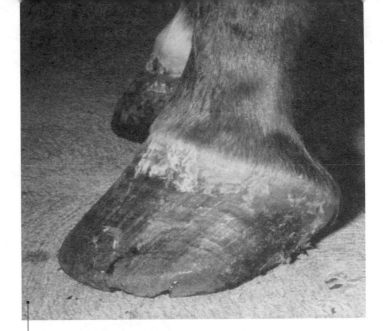

Neglected Bare Hoof
The cause of many hoof problems is neglect. A hoof functions best when it is kept short and in balance, either by natural wear from plenty of exercise or by trimming. When hooves are not trimmed on a regular schedule and in a proper manner, they can grow too long, like this one. The imbalance of a broken-back hoof/pastern angle puts constant excess stress on joints and can lead to navicular syndrome and other serious problems.

Some hoof problems are simply unavoidable accidents, such as stepping on a nail. But many problems, including hoof cracks and lost shoes, are preventable. Almost all problems, large and small, have a better chance of being properly diagnosed, treated, and corrected if you spot them early and take care of them quickly.

Learn how to handle small problems, such as a minor case of thrush, by yourself, but don't hesitate to contact your farrier for advice or assistance. If you find yourself in a situation where you're not sure if something is wrong, or if you know there's a problem but don't know quite what to do about it, your farrier can be a great help.

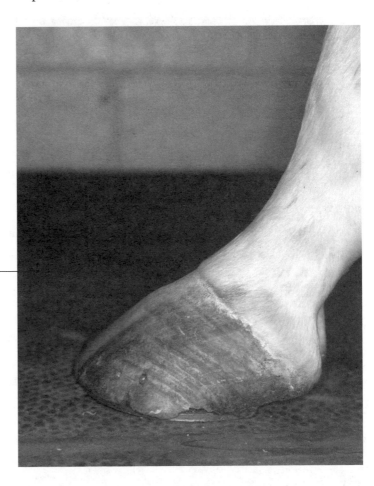

Neglected Shod Hoof
Neglect can lead to problems much more quickly when a horse is shod than when he's barefoot. If you don't ride your horse every day, it's easy to lose track of his shoeing schedule. Make farrier appointments well ahead of time, and mark them on your calendar. This hoof is many weeks overdue and is in serious trouble.

LOST SHOES

Lost shoes are an inconvenience for both the rider and the farrier and can cause hoof damage and lameness. Shoes do not just "fall off," nor does a horse "throw" a shoe. A shoe usually comes off because the horse steps on it or catches it on something, because the hooves are too wet, or because the horse is overdue for shoeing.

Often, the hoof breaks at the time a shoe is lost. Then, while the horse is barefoot, the sole can be bruised and the wall broken further. A shod hoof that is suddenly barefoot is much more susceptible to injury than a hoof that has been conditioned to be barefoot.

Horses commonly lose shoes because they:
- are overdue for shoeing;
- are kept in deep, wet, or muddy footing;
- have an unusual way of moving;
- are subjected to poor balance on the rider's part;
- have abnormal conformation;
- have poor-quality hooves because of inadequate nutrition or poor management;
- have been poorly shod;
- paw;
- have bad luck.

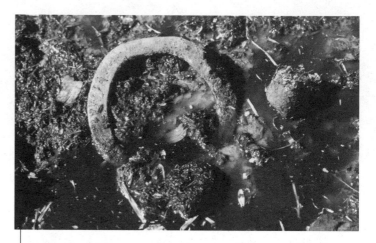

Mud Is a Culprit
Contrary to what many people think, mud does not suck shoes off the hooves of horses. Rather, sticky, slippery mud throws off an animal's balance and timing and makes it more likely that he'll step on and pull off a shoe with another foot. Also, long periods of standing in mud will weaken hoof walls and loosen the hold of the nail clinches.

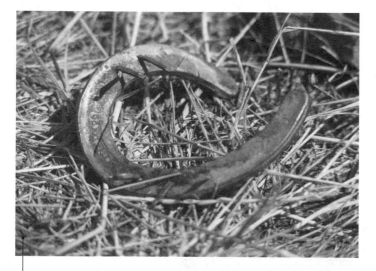

Shoe Stepped Off
If a horse loses a shoe soon after he is shod, it is most likely because he has stepped on it or caught it on something. For this shoe to end up so severely twisted, the horse that lost it was probably moving quite fast when he stepped on it.

Cherry says . . .

THE COST OF A LOST SHOE

A lost shoe costs time, money, and stress. When your horse loses a shoe, it takes time, materials, and effort to protect the bare hoof from damage until the farrier arrives. You might need to trailer the horse to the farrier or make an appointment with the farrier to come to the horse. Getting a shoe replaced might be a matter of hours (not likely), days (hopefully), or weeks (not uncommon).

There is no standard charge for replacing a lost shoe. Some farriers might do it gratis (first one's free), while others might charge you the same amount they would for a full shoeing. If your horse loses a shoe just before a show, a trail ride, or other anticipated event, it can be stressful dealing with the situation and finding someone to replace the shoe quickly. That's one reason to let horses with good hooves go barefoot, to use hoof boots for riding, or to marry a farrier.

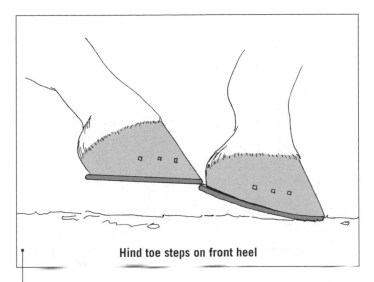

Hind toe steps on front heel

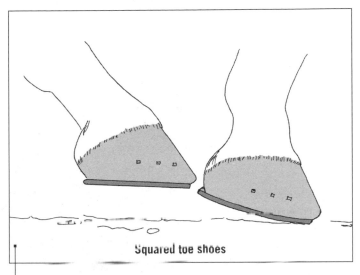

Squared toe shoes

Overreaching: Problem . . .

The toe of a hind shoe can step on the exposed heel of a front shoe and pull it off, the same way you might use the toe of one shoe at the heel of the other to pull off your own shoe. Overreaching is often caused by out-of-balance feet that have delayed breakover and is usually a result of poor shoeing or shoes left on too long.

. . . and Solution

Balancing the feet and using shoes with modified toes that make breakover easier (such as the squared toe shoes shown here) usually prevents a horse from stepping off front shoes. It is tempting to make the heels of the front shoes shorter so they won't be stepped off, but short shoeing can take away necessary support and lead to more serious problems (see page 83).

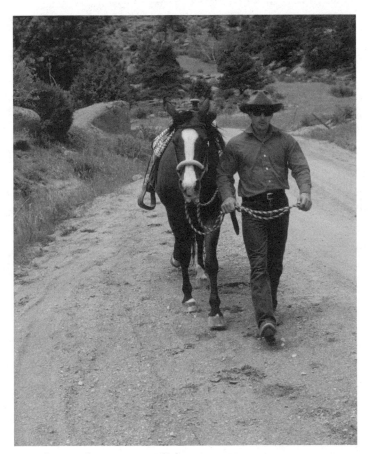

Lost shoe. No boot. Long walk home.

Richard says . . .

DON'T LEAVE HOME WITHOUT IT

If your horse loses a shoe when you're riding in an arena or close to the barn, you can walk him back to his stall or pen, protect the hoof with a wrap or boot, and call the farrier to replace the shoe.

But if Blackie rips off a shoe while you're rounding up strays in the craggy shale beyond the upper leg of Devil's Gulch, riding him home would be like driving a car with a flat tire, not to mention the damage that would be done to his hoof. So make it a rule to pack along a hoof boot that fits your horse whenever you leave the home place. It's always better to have an emergency boot and not need it, than to need one and not have it.

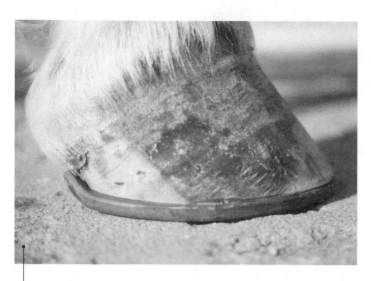

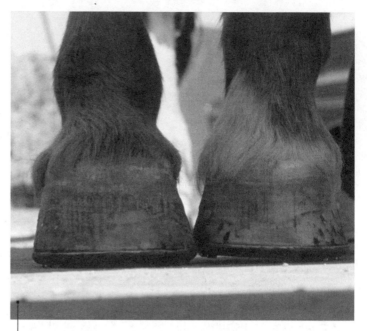

Spooned-Heel Shoe

Horses that have short backs and long legs, or who have developed a quirky way of moving, may continue to step on and pull off front shoes in spite of a farrier's best efforts to balance the feet and ease breakover. Your farrier can make or modify front shoes so the heels angle upward and fit close to the heels of the hoof. This makes it less likely that the toe of a hind hoof will step on the front heel and pull the shoe off.

Stepping on the Opposite Shoe

A horse can also lose a shoe by stepping on the edge of the front shoe with his opposite front foot. This can happen when he's being ridden, while moving over when tied, or when he is turned out.

RICHARD'S CASE NOTES

A Horse That Steps Off Shoes

Scuff marks down the inside of this hind hoof and side clip are evidence that the horse stepped on his opposite hoof many times but did not pull off the shoe.

I shoe this horse's hinds with shoes that have rounded edges on the ground surface and a slight chamfer on the exposed edge of the hoof surface. That way, when the horse steps on his opposite hoof, the rounded shoe edges prevent the shoes from catching and pulling the shoe off.

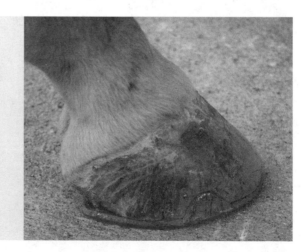

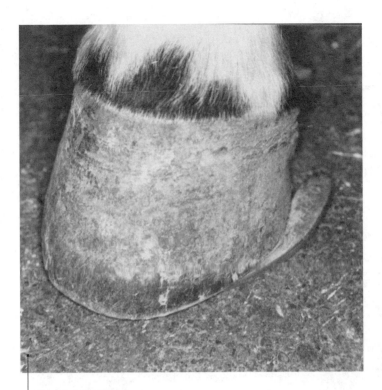

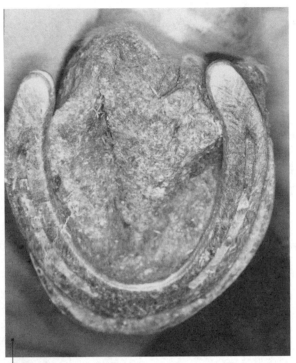

Swiveled Shoe

A shoe can shift or swivel on the hoof when the horse turns or stops quickly, especially if the shoe has a lot of traction. A shoe can also be driven back on a hoof if a horse dances on his hind toes when backing out of a horse trailer or pulls back while tied. A shifted shoe is usually easy to spot because the shoe will stick out farther on one side of the hoof than the other.

Reset a Shifted Shoe

A shifted shoe will usually not stay on long, and it is a danger because it could cut the opposite leg. It should be reset as soon as possible. If the shoe is very loose, remove it and protect the hoof until the farrier arrives (see pages 88–92). If the shoe is still tight, keep the horse confined until it can be reset.

Sprung Shoe

A sprung shoe has one bent heel and is no longer flat or level. This usually happens when a horse steps on the heel of the shoe with another foot or catches the shoe on a fence or other object. Even though the shoe still might be firmly attached, a sprung shoe will put uneven stress on the hoof and should be removed, straightened, and reset as soon as possible.

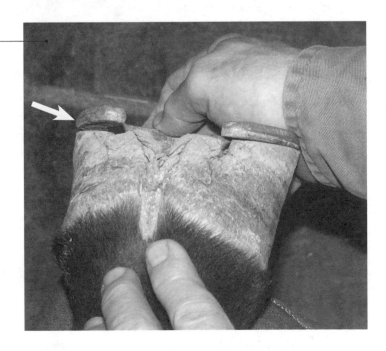

Buddy Solves the Lost Shoe Mystery

Since the beginning of my career I've kept detailed records of the horses I shoe. For every horse, I have recorded hoof measurements, the owner's shoe preferences, and the horse's grade during shoeing. I also note how often a horse loses a shoe and which shoe it was. Looking at this data, I know that the average shoe loss of all my clients is 1.33 shoes per horse per year, that 80 percent of all lost shoes can be attributed to 20 percent of the horses, and that within that 20 percent group a certain few horses lost most of the shoes.

Now, it has always been my policy to replace a horse's first lost shoe free of charge. After that first time, the owner pays a flat service charge, plus hoof-repair costs, if needed.

Bob and Laurie were new to the area, and their big sorrel gelding, Buster, was a real stinker. Not that he was bad to shoe. No, he stood like a gentleman with Buddy, his yellow Lab pal, lying politely nearby, waiting for trimmings to chew. The problem was that Buster lost three shoes the first week I worked on him.

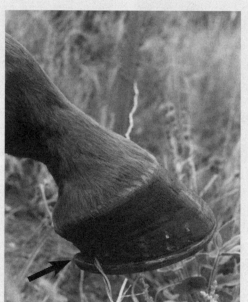

On the first lost-shoe call, Bob and Laurie were amazed that I showed up the same day they called and were very pleased with my standard "first one is free" policy.

"Well, lost shoes happen," I said, and since they hadn't found the lost shoe, I applied a new shoe and was soon on my way.

Two days later I was back. Same hoof, right front, shoe not found. Luckily, Buster had sturdy hooves, and both shoes had come off clean. He lived in a smooth wire paddock of soft dirt, so his bare hoof wasn't damaged.

Bob and Laurie watched quietly as I put on my apron, and I sensed a creeping shadow of doubt in my competence. I applied another new shoe, charged the flat fee this time, and was on to my next appointment.

Three days later I awoke to a curt early-morning phone message.

"Buster threw the same shoe again."

Now, I knew he hadn't "thrown" it, and his conformation was such that he likely wasn't stepping the shoes off, either. I had a hunch what Buster's problem was, but I needed one of the lost shoes to prove it. Buddy helped me clinch it.

When I pulled into the drive, Buddy was sitting pleased as punch. The Lab had found the lost shoe, one of the three, and deposited it on the back porch like a trophy, six nails straight up. Some kind of good retriever. I examined the shoe, as Bob and Laurie stood with folded arms looking somewhat grim.

As I'd suspected, the hoof surface edge of one heel was shiny from the end to the last nail (see arrow). I pulled the nails, cleaned the shoe, and nailed it through the old familiar holes in Buster's hoof. As Bob returned Buster to his pen, I asked Laurie, "You haven't seen Buster pawing the fence, have you?"

"Oh, no. Buster's never done that," she replied defensively. Bob chimed in as he joined us, "Maybe you just need to use a smaller shoe or more nails, like our last shoer did."

I was inhaling a head of steam to launch my "Lost Shoes Are a Fact of Life" presentation when the fence behind us began shaking. We all three turned to see Buster, 50 feet down the fence line, with the heel of his right front shoe securely hooked on the bottom wire.

HOOF CRACKS

A crack is a horizontal or vertical break in the hoof wall. Horizontal cracks are called blowouts. Vertical cracks are referred to by their location at the toe, quarters, and heels. Vertical cracks that originate at the coronet are called sand cracks, while those that start at the ground surface are called grass cracks.

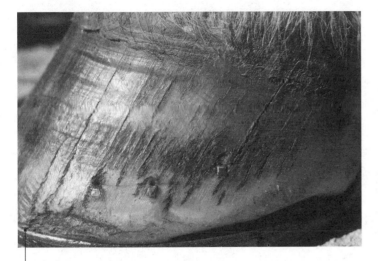

Surface Cracks

Surface cracks are superficial fissures that cover varying portions of the hoof wall. They are usually caused by a change in hoof moisture, such as when a horse on wet pasture is put in a stall with dry bedding or when a horse who has been standing in mud then stands in the sunshine. Prevention and treatment of surface cracks are the same:

- Make sure the horse is getting a balanced diet for optimum hoof health.
- Stabilize the horse's hoof-moisture balance.
- Minimize exposure to wet footing.
- Apply a hoof sealer or hardener.

When treating a surface crack, keep in mind that a hoof dressing might fill the cracks and improve the appearance of a hoof, but a hoof sealer or hardener will be more beneficial to long-term hoof health.

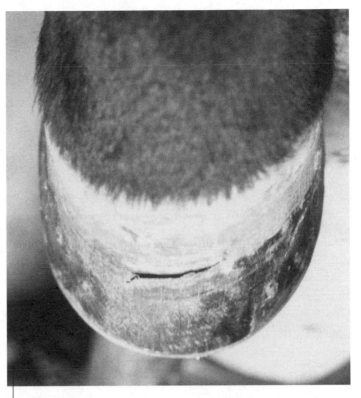

Blowout

A horizontal crack in the hoof wall is called a blowout. Blowouts are caused either by an injury to the coronary band or by a blow to the hoof wall (see page 34). A blowout usually will not result in lameness, and many times will go unnoticed until the farrier spots it. Once it occurs, a blowout will seldom increase in size and will usually require no treatment. However, a blowout can set the stage for a vertical crack if the hoof is weakened by excess moisture or if hoof balance is not maintained.

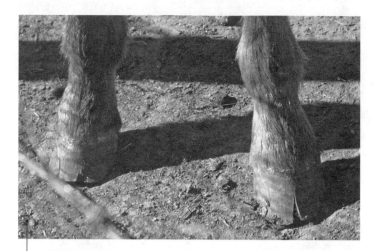

Grass Crack

Grass cracks appear most often in neglected, unshod hooves. A hoof that is allowed to grow too long will usually break off in chunks at the quarters and often crack from the ground up at the toe.

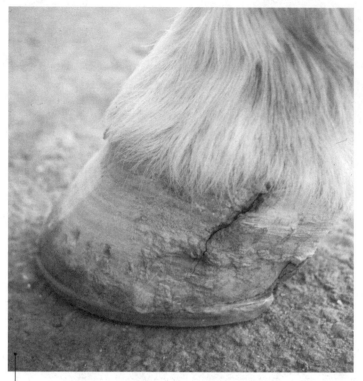

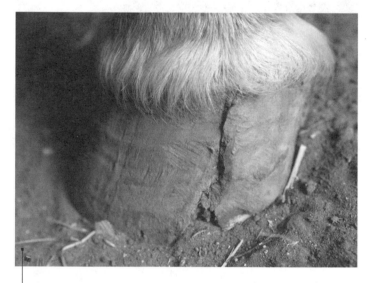

Full Crack

If a small crack is not addressed, it can become a full crack that runs the length of the hoof. This is a serious problem that usually causes extreme pain and lameness.

Sand Crack

A sand crack, or high quarter crack, is a vertical crack that can result from an imbalanced hoof, extreme stress, injury to the coronet, or an infection in the foot that breaks out at the coronet. An imbalanced hoof can overload the quarter of the hoof where the hoof wall is thinnest and result in a crack. High-impact activities such as racing and jumping can put extreme stress on the hoof and cause a high quarter crack. Sometimes a horse will hit the opposite hoof during fast work or an uncoordinated movement. This can set the stage for a sand crack. A wet environment can soften a horse's hooves and allow particles of sand or gravel to be forced up into the white line. If infection results, it can travel upward through the laminae and break out at the coronet, causing a crack to form.

CRACK TREATMENT

A crack does not "heal," but must be replaced by new growth from the coronary band, just as a damaged fingernail must grow out. This will take between nine and twelve months. For optimal hoof growth, it is essential that the horse's ration contain nutrients necessary for healthy hooves (see page 30).

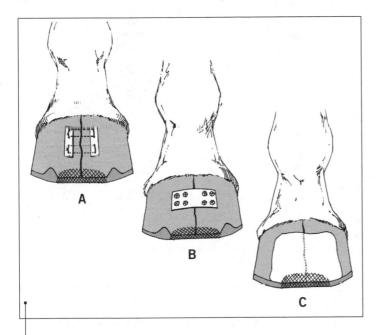

Toe-Crack Treatments

Severe cracks may need to be held immobile and perhaps shod until new hoof grows down and replaces the cracked area. Methods for stabilizing a crack include:

A. drilling holes on either side of the crack and using fine wire or some other material to lace up the crack like a boot;

B. fastening a metal plate across the crack with screws;

C. gluing a patch over the crack.

Special hoof-repair adhesives mimic the consistency of the hoof wall, can withstand the pressure of driven nails, and can be trimmed and rasped along with the hoof wall as it grows down.

Before a crack is stabilized using any method, it must be thoroughly cleansed of dirt, loose hoof horn, and bacteria. If there is any evidence of moist-sensitive tissue, the crack should be treated by a veterinarian until it is completely dry. Applying a patch over a moist crack without leaving access for flushing and draining the area leads to infection.

The first step in dealing with a crack is to determine the cause and remove it. Often, all that is needed to control and treat a toe crack is a good, balanced trim that carefully rounds the edges of the hoof. Especially with toe cracks, it is essential that proper hoof angle be maintained in order to minimize stress on the hoof at the toe as the crack grows out. A squared toe shoe can reduce the prying effect of breakover at the front of the hoof.

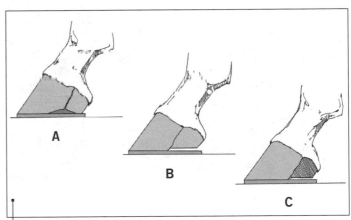

Quarter-Crack Treatment

Like toe cracks, quarter cracks can be laced with wire or other suture material. This method is risky and requires a great deal of skill because the hoof wall is typically very thin at the quarters. There are other treatments that do not require holding the crack together. One method **(A)** requires the farrier to "relieve" or pare away the cracked portion of the hoof on either side of the crack so it doesn't touch the shoe or bear weight. Depending on the crack, it may be patched as with a toe crack in the previous illustration.

Another approach to quarter-crack treatment **(B)** calls for application of a full-support shoe (see page 62) and "floating" the portion of the hoof behind the crack. To float a heel means to trim the heel about ¼ inch (0.64 cm) shorter so it will not touch the shoe. By eliminating weight bearing behind the crack, movement of the two halves of the crack is minimized and the hoof has a better chance of growing down intact.

The most intensive treatment for very severe or chronic quarter cracks **(C)** involves removing (resecting) the area of the hoof wall behind the crack. A full-support shoe is applied until new hoof grows to ground level.

RICHARD'S CASE NOTES

Crack Treatment, Before and After

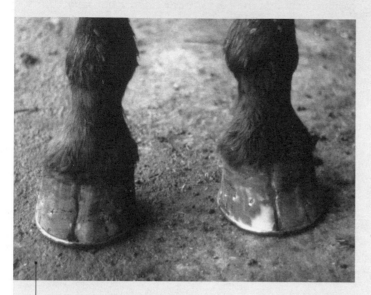

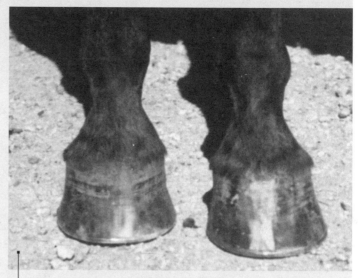

Chronic Toe Cracks

The first time that I shod this horse's fronts, he had very wide toe cracks running from the coronet to the ground, which the owner said had been present for many years. I balanced the feet and shod them with plain shoes. The cracks were not patched or filled. I put the horse on my schedule and suggested the owner apply hoof sealer daily and keep the horse on dry footing as much as possible.

Fourteen Months Later

The owner was diligent about applying hoof sealer regularly, keeping her horse on dry footing when possible, and sticking to a six-week shoeing schedule. These three steps were all it took. Within one year and two months, her horse had grown new, solid front hooves.

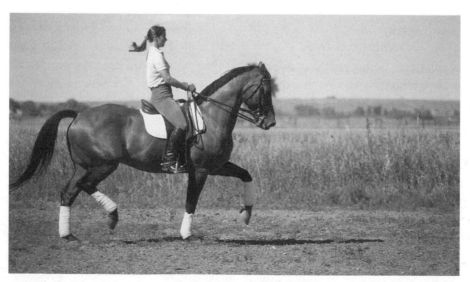

Don't let cracks or thrush put your horse out of commission.

THRUSH TREATMENT

Thrush is caused by bacteria that thrive in the warm, dark recesses of the hoof, usually the clefts of the frog. Many horses have lesser degrees of thrush that require no treatment other than periodic hoof cleaning. However, in some cases, thrush can invade sensitive tissues and cause lameness. Thrush can also invade separations and cracks in a hoof wall, especially if a horse is constantly on wet footing.

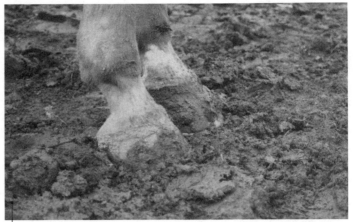

Recipe for Thrush
Horses, especially those in confinement, often don't have a dry place to stand, and even if they do, for comfort they often choose to stand in soft wet bedding, manure, or mud, at least part of the time. Wet footing almost always results in thrush.

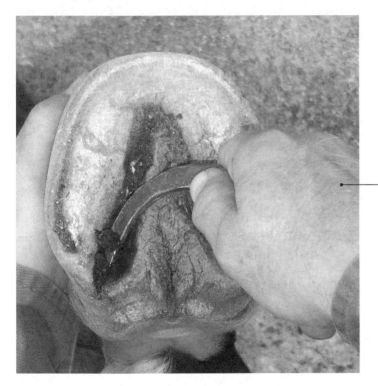

Thrush Evidence
It's easy to tell if your horse has thrush. When you clean the clefts of the frog, the evidence is a white cheesy or foul-smelling black gook you'll see on your hoof pick. Once you've smelled it, you'll never mistake it. Thrush bacteria are anaerobic, which means they thrive in areas sealed off from oxygen (air). The best way to avoid thrush is to keep your horse's feet clean and dry so air can reach the tissues.

SUGARDINE

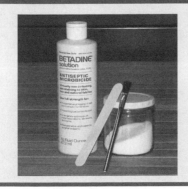

Sugardine is a homemade thrush remedy that's effective and easy to use; it doesn't stain, has no bad odor, and is inexpensive. Sugardine has been used for years in human medicine to treat wounds and burns. It reduces edema (swelling), nourishes surface cells, and speeds healing. To make sugardine, mix povidone-iodine (Betadine) with granulated sugar to form a thin paste. Generic povidone-iodine is often half the price of Betadine and is basically the same product.

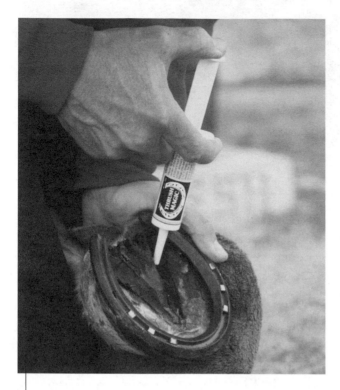

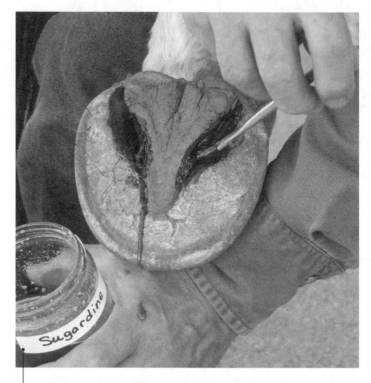

Thrush Remedies

Commercial thrush remedies are available in liquids, pastes, and creams and vary in effectiveness, ease of use, and cost. Some products are preventives when used regularly, while others are designed to cure thrush after it is established. Applicators vary from spray and squirt bottles to syringes and brushes. Some applicators make it easy to inject the product into the clefts without making a mess.

While the purple or green color of some liquid products lets you see your application clearly, these products can stain everything they touch, including clothes, hands, and your horse's clean white socks.

Never use bleach or hydrogen peroxide on thrush. These chemicals can destroy healthy tissues of the frog and can actually retard healing.

Applying Sugardine

1. First, trim away loose and overgrown flaps of the frog using a sharp hoof knife, to allow air and the medication to reach the affected tissues. If you're not comfortable doing this, ask your farrier or vet for help.
2. Wash the hoof thoroughly with mild soap, such as Betadine scrub, and plenty of warm water.
3. Pat the hoof dry with a cloth, and apply sugardine deep into the clefts of the frog using a small brush. An acid brush, available at hardware stores, has short, flat, black bristles and a 6-inch-long (15.2 cm) tubular metal handle and is effective for this purpose.
4. Stir the sugardine thoroughly before each use, as the sugar will settle to the bottom of the container.
5. Apply sugardine daily until the thrush is gone.
6. Keep the horse's feet as clean and dry as possible to speed healing and prevent recurrence.

LONG TOE/LOW HEEL

A long toe and low heel (LT/LH) hoof configuration is the number-one cause of hoof problems. When a hoof becomes too low in the heel and the hoof pastern axis is broken backwards, it puts constant excess stress on the foot, especially on the flexor tendon and the navicular bone. This restricts blood flow within the foot, causes heel soreness, cracks, contracted heels, and navicular syndrome; and it can lead to irreversible changes in the hoof structure.

Hoof Angle Review

The angle of normal healthy hooves is typically between 52 and 60 degrees. A line through the center of the pastern will be roughly parallel to the front surface of the coffin bone. In a healthy, well-formed hoof with no flares, the front of the hoof wall is parallel to the front of the coffin bone. (See pages 3 and 82.)

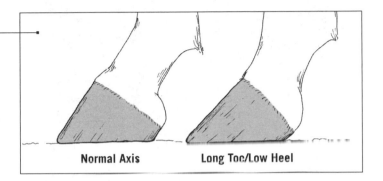

Normal Axis   **Long Toe/Low Heel**

RICHARD'S CASE NOTES

Extreme Long Toe/Low Heel

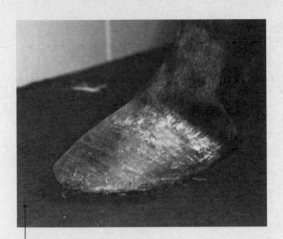

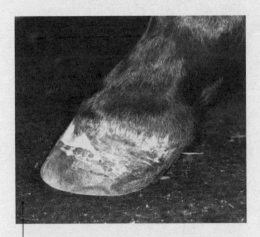

Before Trimming

Like many domestic horses, this brood mare was confined on soft footing with very little exercise. Consequently, her hooves grew faster than they could wear away. Since hooves angle forward, the longer they grow, the more weight is put on the heels. This overload causes heels to grow more slowly than the toe. Because the owner neglected to have the feet trimmed regularly, his horse developed LT/LH. When the horse was brought to the vet clinic, she showed obvious discomfort when walking on a lead and was reluctant to trot.

After Trimming

Fortunately, the mare had good-quality hooves, and, by trimming once, I was able to restore hoof angles to normal without the use of shoes or pads. She now moved out much more freely but continued to show slight lameness on the fronts at the trot. The vet suspected navicular damage, but the owner declined to have further testing done and didn't want the horse shod.

Consistent trimming by a professional farrier can prevent LT/LH from occurring. And like this horse, many that are suffering discomfort show immediate improvement once their hooves are properly trimmed.

Shoes Left On Too Long

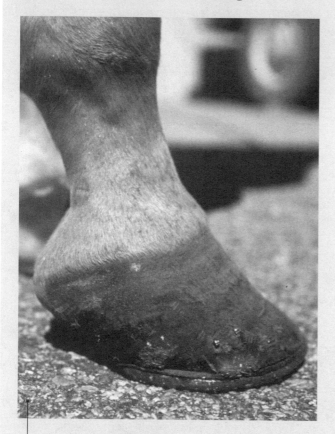

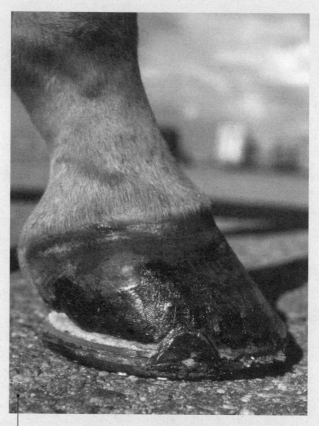

Long Toe/Low Heel

Leaving shoes on a horse too long will almost always result in LT/LH. This horse was so uncomfortable with his low hoof angles that he could not be ridden. Even though his hooves might have been balanced properly when he was shod, the shoes were left on way too long. Once the heels expanded over the shoes, the heels collapsed while the toe continued to grow longer and developed a dish.

After a Trim and New Shoes

In some cases, such as when the heels are crushed, there will not be enough hoof for the farrier to work with to restore proper angle and alignment by trimming alone. This horse was immediately more comfortable after trimming. Wedge pads were initially required to restore normal hoof angles. After the next shoeing cycle (shown here), he was shod with flat pads and was back to his previous level of performance.

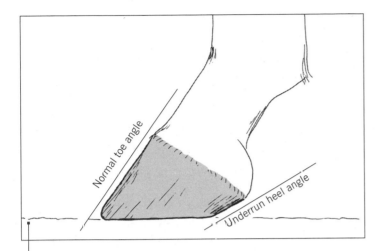

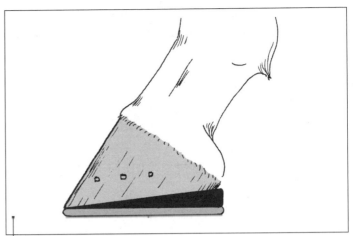

Underrun Heels

A common result of LT/LH is underrun heels. This is an often-irreversible condition where the angle of the hoof horn at the heel is lower than the angle at the toe by 5 degrees or more. The hoof wall at the heel angles forward and "runs under" the hoof. This puts the natural base of support provided by the hoof too far forward under the hoof. Underrun heels can be difficult, if not impossible, to correct.

Trimming Underrun Heels

To correct underrun heels, a farrier first must trim the horse's heels short. This does two things: It transfers support for the hoof rearward, where it belongs, and it reduces the crushing leverage that the horse's weight puts on long underrun heels. If the hoof angle is too low once the heels are trimmed, a wedge shoe or wedge pad, as illustrated here, can be used to bring the angle up to normal.

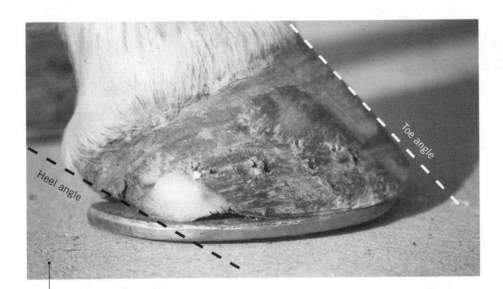

Shoeing Underrun Heels

There are two things your farrier can do that will really improve LT/LH and underrun heels. He can use a modified toe shoe to ease breakover (see page 63), and he can use extended heels or an egg bar shoe to be sure the shoe extends behind the hoof for maximum support. This underrun hoof is shod with a squared toe, extended-heel shoe.

Despite the best care, some underrun heels never return to normal. But with proper trimming and shoeing, the horse can be made comfortable and usable.

CONTRACTED HEELS

When the heels of a hoof contract (shrink or move closer together), they can put pressure on the inner parts of the hoof and cause lameness.

Causes of Contracted Heels

- **Long toe/low heel.** When the horse's weight rotates over a long toe, the heels of the hoof are drawn inward.
- **Non–weight bearing.** When the horse does not put any weight on the foot, such as when the limb is recovering from an injury.
- **Lack of exercise.** When a horse is confined to a stall or his exercise is otherwise restricted. The majority of moisture in a hoof comes from the blood, and without exercise, blood flow in the foot is decreased, and the hoof dries out and curls inward.
- **Physical restriction.** When the hoof is in a cast or bandage.
- **Poor shoeing.** When nails or clips are applied too far back on the hoof; generally, nails should not be used behind the widest part of the foot.

Treatment of Contracted Heels

The first step in the treatment of contracted heels is to identify the cause and remove it. A foot that has contracted from being in a cast, for example, will usually return to normal health once the cast is off and the horse gets regular exercise.

Simply balancing a contracted hoof that has long toe/low heel will allow the hoof to function more normally and will encourage the heels to spread. The horse can be left barefoot, if practical, or can be shod with a squared toe shoe with adequate heel support. In some instances, a frog-support pad or a shoe similar to a heart bar shoe is applied in order to stimulate blood flow within the hoof.

Once the horse has adequate exercise, blood flow in the foot will increase and make the hoof wall suppler. If the horse is too sore to exercise, the hoof can be soaked in a boot, wrapped with wet bandages, and the horse bedded in damp sand or sawdust to increase hoof moisture and make the hoof more pliable. Once a normal moisture level has been attained and the horse is exercising, a hoof sealer can be applied to prevent internal moisture from evaporating through the hoof wall.

There are various mechanical devices and shoes used to physically spread the heels of a contracted hoof, but efforts to employ these tools will be futile unless you first remove the cause of the contraction.

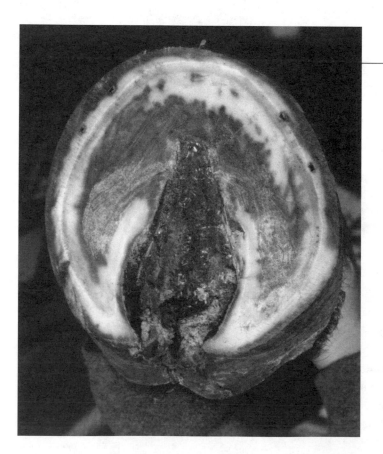

Contracted Heel Fix

The heels of this hoof appear to have contracted; the heels are pointing towards the frog instead of pointing rearward. In a case like this, if the horse is sound, there is no need for special measures to expand the heels. Simply make sure the foot is balanced and, if shoes are applied, be sure they do not restrict expansion at the heels.

Cherry says . . .

DON'T CRAMP HER STYLE

The horses I've seen with contracted heels, such as young halter horses, remind me of a woman wearing a pair of high-heeled shoes that are too small and too tight. Luckily, with a good farrier and plenty of regular exercise, contracted heels are reversible.

MISMATCHED HOOVES

When a horse has one small, upright front hoof and another that is slightly larger with a lower heel, he is said to have "mismatched" or "high/low" hooves. This condition can affect any breed; it is usually established when a horse is young, and it can stay that way for life.

High/low hooves can be caused by the way a foal stands to graze, with one front foot consistently forward and the other foot always back underneath him. When the foal constantly assumes this grazing position, the heel of the hoof thrust forward becomes low and the hoof of the foot that's set back becomes steep. Mismatched hooves might also be caused by an injury or soreness that causes a foal to bear weight unevenly on his front feet for an extended period.

Mild high/low hooves, when the difference between them is one shoe size or an angle of less than 3 degrees, can usually be trimmed so that angles match and the hooves take the same size shoe.

When the angles of the hooves differ by more than 3 degrees, it is sometimes better to change them only conservatively and let the angles be somewhat different. This is because mismatched hooves can affect the alignment of the legs, shoulders, and even the spine of a horse. Making radical changes in hoof angles, in an effort to make them match, might cause problems elsewhere.

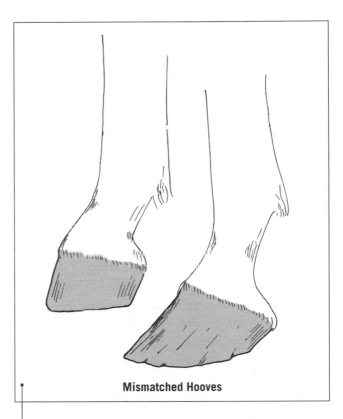

Mismatched Hooves

Mismatched hooves can be slight or dramatic; may or may not cause lameness; might be okay as is or require specialized trimming or shoeing.

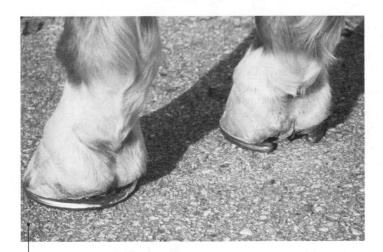

It's Okay to Be Different

For balanced movement and an even stride, it may be necessary to outfit a horse with two different front shoes. A horse might wear a squared toe egg bar on the low hoof and a full-toed plain shoe on the steep hoof. The egg bar provides support for the low heels, and the squared toe will help speed breakover to match that of the steeper hoof.

Richard says . . .

BALANCE FOR MOVEMENT

Some horse owners and some shoers get hung up on the idea that a horse's feet should be matched pairs. For example, they might believe that the right front should be identical to the left front in size and shape.

As a general rule this is true, the hooves will match. But an experienced farrier will often shoe the horse for balanced movement rather than for balanced appearance. Sometimes to help a horse move better the feet will be trimmed and shod differently from one another. It's better to have a sound horse with mismatched feet than a lame horse with matching feet.

STUMBLING

A horse that stumbles is risky to ride, since you never know when he is suddenly going to fall out from under you. Any horse can trip occasionally, but a consistent stumbler is dangerous. Take time to find the cause of the stumbling, and discuss remedies with your farrier.

Causes and Solutions

OVERDUE HOOF CARE. *Waiting too long to schedule trimming or shoeing leads to long toe/low heel imbalance, which throws off the timing of a horse's stride. A long toe is more likely than a shorter toe to cause tripping on uneven footing.*

SOLUTION: Have your horse trimmed regularly to keep his hooves in balance.

POOR CONDITION. *A young horse or a horse that's been out of work may stumble because he's out of shape.*

SOLUTION: Use a progressive conditioning program to develop a young horse or bring a seasoned horse back into work after a layoff. Develop the horse's entire physique so he is light on his forehand and carries appropriate weight on his hindquarters.

FATIGUE. *A tired horse is more likely to stumble than a horse that's fresh.*

SOLUTION: Get your horse in shape, and stop working him when he gets tired. Squared toe and rocker toe shoes make each step easier. With these shoes a horse can travel longer without tiring, and when he does get fatigued, they reduce the chance of stumbling. They are especially effective for endurance horses.

RIDER ERROR. *An inexperienced, uncoordinated, or inattentive rider can throw a horse off balance and cause him to stumble. In order to shift his weight rearward to stay balanced, a horse must be able to raise and lower his head and neck.*

SOLUTION: Try not to restrict your horse's head movement by improper use of reins, tie-downs, or other means. Have your riding evaluated by an experienced riding instructor, and get yourself in shape so you can maintain a proper position when riding.

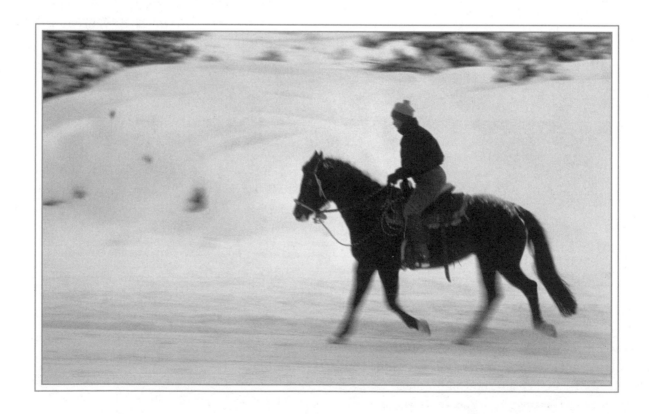

WAYS OF GOING. *A horse that travels heavy on the forehand is more likely to stumble than one that carries more of his weight on the hindquarters. Rope walking can also cause stumbling. That happens when a horse places one foot directly in front of the other and stumbles over his own feet.*

SOLUTION: Train your horse to be lighter on his forehand by working to develop natural collection (see the Resource Guide for recommended reading on the topic of horse training). Shoeing techniques that encourage a horse to break over the center of his hooves or slightly to the outside can help counteract rope walking.

ATTITUDE AND ATTENTION. *A lazy or bored horse that doesn't pick up his feet is more likely to stumble than a horse that is alert and energetic.*

SOLUTION: Don't let the horse fall into a zoned-out or mechanical mode. Vary your riding and training workouts, and make sure you're paying attention, too.

SHOEING PROBLEM. *A shoeing style that starts out with low heels and long toes or uses shoes that are too small can cause stumbling.*

SOLUTION: Have the horse's shoeing evaluated by a qualified farrier. Trimming the hooves into balance might be all that's required to solve the problem. If your present farrier can't or won't work with you to fix the problem, find one who will.

PHYSICAL PROBLEMS. *Any condition anywhere on the body that limits a horse's awareness or movement or causes him pain is a possible cause of stumbling. These include sore heels, a painful tooth or neck, navicular syndrome, and arthritis.*

SOLUTION: If traditional veterinary procedures fail to uncover or alleviate stumbling, you might consider having the horse examined by an equine chiropractor or acupuncturist.

ILL-FITTING TACK. *Inappropriate or poorly fitted tack can cause the horse pain or discomfort, leading to poor movement and stumbling.*

SOLUTION: Check to see if the saddle might be pinching the horse's withers or if the saddle skirts are hitting his hips. Make sure the bit is not pinching the skin at the corners of his mouth and that the headstall fits correctly. Be sure support boots fit properly, are clean, and are not too tight. Check that hoof boots are not chafing his pastern or coronet. Make sure the cinch is not hitting the horse's elbow. Check the cinch and saddle blanket for burrs and other objects before tacking up.

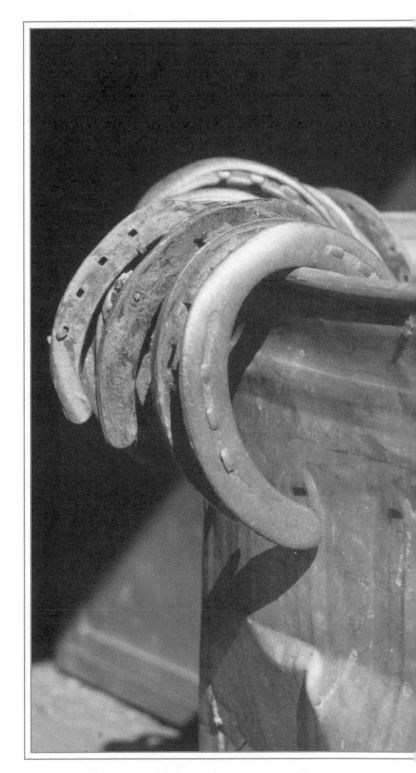

FORGING AND OVERREACHING

Forging and overreaching are two gait defects that involve contact between the hind and the front feet. A horse that forges or overreaches may be more prone to stumble or fall, especially if the heel of the front shoe is stepped on. Forging and overreaching are indications that the horse's movement is out of balance.

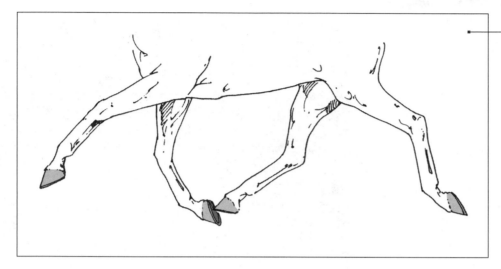

Forging

Forging occurs when the toe of the hind hoof or shoe hits the front hoof or shoe on the same side of the horse. This usually happens at a trot and makes a characteristic *click-click* sound if the horse is shod or a softer *thup-thup* if the horse is barefoot. A horse can get front-sole bruises from forging.

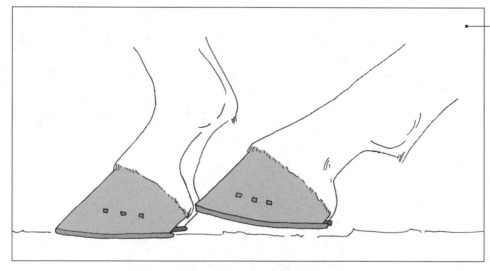

Overreaching

Overreaching happens when the hind hoof or shoe hits part of the front foot, such as the heel, bulb, coronary band, fetlock, or flexor tendon. This often results in injury.

Causes of Forging and Overreaching

- Imbalanced hooves. This is usually long toe/low heel on fronts, hinds, or all.
- Poor conditioning of the horse. A horse that's out of shape will not move as athletically or with as much balance as a horse that is fit.
- Fatigue. A tired horse will tend to move in a sloppy manner.
- Poor riding. The rider is not balanced on the horse or is not keeping the horse collected and moving energetically.
- Sore-footedness or lameness. Uncomfortable feet can throw off a horse's timing and rhythm.
- Soft, deep, or wet footing can unbalance a horse and cause him to move erratically.

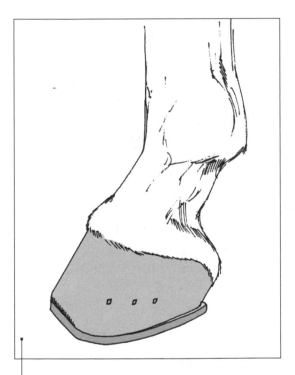

Squared Toe Shoes Can Prevent Overreaching and Forging

Assuming the habits and techniques associated with the health care, conditioning, training, and riding of your horse have been evaluated and changed if necessary, trimming and shoeing may be able to help eliminate forging or overreaching. Restoring a horse's normal hoof configuration and balance is often all that is needed to enable a horse to trot freely without forging or overreaching. If the problem persists, however, easing breakover on all four feet by using modified-toe shoes, such as squared toes, will usually solve the problem.

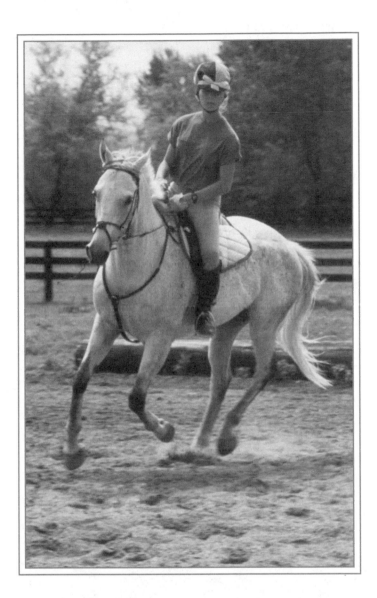

Richard says . . .

A NEAR SURE CURE

No matter what is causing a horse to forge or overreach, I've found that balancing the hooves and applying squared toe shoes all around will fix the problem in most cases. Squaring the toe of a shoe is an easy modification that can even be done cold by a farrier skilled with a hammer. This can be a simple solution to an annoying problem. (See page 99.)

INTERFERING

Interfering occurs when a horse hits the inside of his leg or foot with the opposite hoof. It can occur between the knee and the hoof of the front limbs and between the hock and the hoof of the hind limbs. Often both legs of a pair are affected — the right hind strikes the left hind and the left hind strikes the right hind. Interfering rarely occurs at the walk. It appears most commonly at the trot, at the canter, and when backing. The speed and energy level with which a horse moves his limbs can affect the tendency to interfere. For example, a horse may interfere at a lazy jog but not at an energetic extended trot, or vice versa.

Causes of Interfering

As with forging, interfering can have many causes, and you might have to play Sherlock to figure out a solution.

Conformation. Interfering of the fronts is frequently associated with narrow-chested and/or toed-out horses. A narrow chest places the limbs closer together, and the toed-out hoof tends to make the leg swing inward when the horse moves.

Horse imbalance. Interfering often occurs simply because the horse is trying to keep his balance. He is attempting to keep his limbs under his center of mass.

Basically, there are three forces at work when a horse moves: the vertical force of the weight of the horse and rider; the horizontal force of the horse moving forward; and the swinging or side-to-side motion of the horse at various gaits. Exactly where under his body a horse places his limbs is determined in large part by the interaction of these three forces and the direction of their composite. A barefoot horse moving freely in a pasture rarely interferes. It is when he carries a rider and is asked to perform in collected and extended frames and at both faster and slower speeds that interfering occurs.

Hoof imbalance. If a hoof is obviously imbalanced, then trimming (and shoeing if necessary) should be the first step to correcting interfering. If the hooves are balanced and the horse is still interfering, then riding, conditioning, and training should be evaluated and changed if needed before turning to corrective shoes.

Shoeing techniques include modifying shoes to direct the hooves to break over a specific part of the toe, applying a shoe so it lines up with the horse's midline rather than with the hoof, and setting the shoe off-center on the hoof, so the base of support is directly under the horse's leg. Foot flight, the way the foot moves past the opposite leg, can be affected by lowering one side of a hoof and by the use of side-weighted shoes. When shoeing to correct interfering, experimentation over a period of time that includes a number of farrier visits is often necessary. Trimming and shoeing alterations should be approached conservatively and monitored closely to ensure that joints in a horse's legs are not being unduly stressed.

Cuts and Bruises from Interfering

If a horse does not wear protective boots, the first signs of interfering may be pain, heat, or swelling in the area of contact. The problem may escalate to include missing hair, bruises, cuts, lesions, chronic sores, and, perhaps, underlying bone damage.

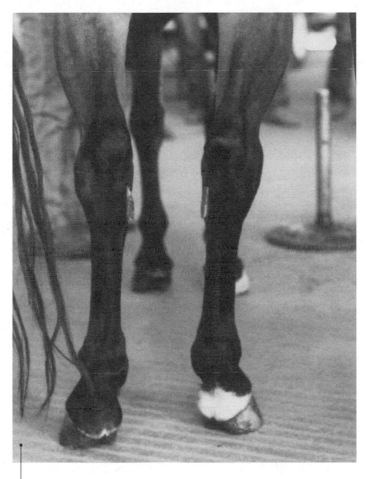

Toed-Out Hinds
Interfering between the hind legs is often associated with a toed-out conformation.

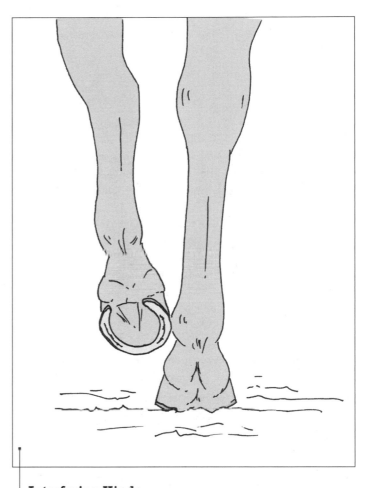

Interfering Hinds
Some horses will continue to interfere in spite of the best management, riding, training, and farrier care.

Changing the Breakover Point
A farrier can modify a shoe so that it encourages the hoof to break over a specific part of the toe in order to prevent interfering. The goal is to have the leg travel straight forward rather than swinging inward where it might hit the opposite leg.

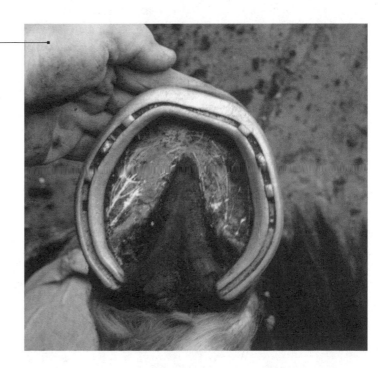

-12-
CALL THE
VET

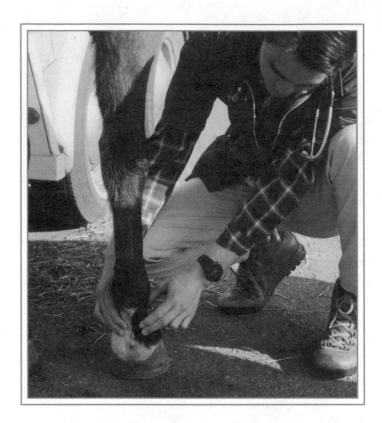

S ome hoof problems require veterinary care along with therapeutic shoeing. Knowing how your vet will likely want to approach serious hoof problems will make you better able to assist in your horse's treatment and to monitor his recovery.

BRUISES

Like your own feet, the soles of your horse's feet become conditioned to the type of ground he lives on. A horse with flat or soft soles that have little or no protective layer of callus, or whose soles have been worn or trimmed too thin, may move timidly on gravel or other rough surfaces. The underlying layer of sensitive sole can bruise easily when he steps on stones or frozen ground. These bruises are seldom visible right away because they are beneath the outer sole. However, they are sensitive immediately to hoof testers and sometimes even to heavy thumb pressure.

Later, when the sole is trimmed, the bruise will be evident. A dry bruise appears dark or red; a wet bruise leaks serum. Infected bruises are serious because the infection could spread to the laminae or to a bone or joint.

If recent trimming resulted in a thin sole, the horse may be off and "ouchy" even when shod. Until the sole grows thick enough for the horse to be comfortable, a hoof boot can protect hooves while the horse is worked or ridden. This is usually necessary only for a week or two.

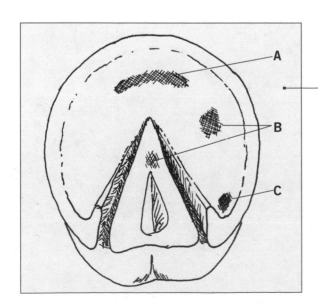

Where Bruises Occur
Bruises are most commonly found in the following places for the following reasons:
A. Crescent-shaped bruises at the toe are usually caused by the sensitive sole being compressed between the hard outer sole and the front edge of the coffin bone.
B. Bruises at the toe, quarter areas of the sole, and on the frog are often caused by stones or lumpy frozen ground.
C. A bruise in the buttress (corn) is usually due to contact with a stone, pressure from an improperly applied shoe, or a shoe that's left on too long.

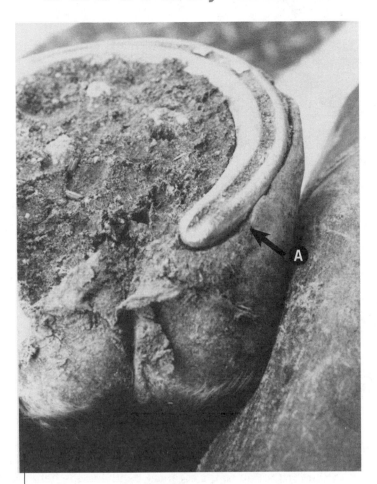

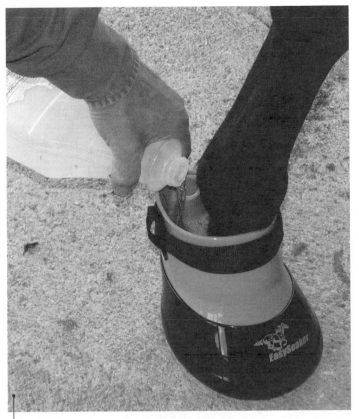

Overgrown Shoes Can Cause Corns

A corn is a bruise at the buttress where the hoof wall curves to join the bars. This site is actually called the seat of corn. Corns are typically caused by pressure from an overgrown horseshoe or from a stone that's become wedged between the shoe and the hoof. When the hoof is trimmed, the seat of corn should be pared below the level of the hoof wall to prevent its contact with the shoe. When a hoof overgrows the shoe, the heels of the hoof often collapse and the shoe presses on the seat of corn **(A)**, resulting in a bruise.

A corn can cause varying degrees of lameness. Trimming the hoof to remove pressure on the corn may be the only treatment required. But if the corn is infected, it must be treated as an abscess.

Treatment of Bruises and Abscesses

Treatment of a hoof abscess involves three steps: paring, soaking, and protecting. Typically, your vet will pare away the sole around the abscess so it can drain. Then the foot is soaked in an antiseptic solution. Your vet may perform all of the tasks or may entrust you with the daily soaking and wrapping.

Using a soaking boot might be easier than trying to get your horse to stand with his foot in a bucket. Put the boot on a clean hoof and pour warm water into the top of the boot. After soaking, the foot is dried and bandaged to keep the wound clean. Applying a hoof boot over the bandage provides additional protection to the tender sole and prevents wear on the bandage. Soaking and wrapping is often done daily.

A treatment-plate shoe (see page 60) eliminates the need for bandaging, requires only a small amount of medicated packing, and provides absolute protection to the sole. A treatment-plate shoe will cost more than a boot, and finding a farrier who can make and apply the shoe might be difficult, but you'll save significantly in bandaging time and materials.

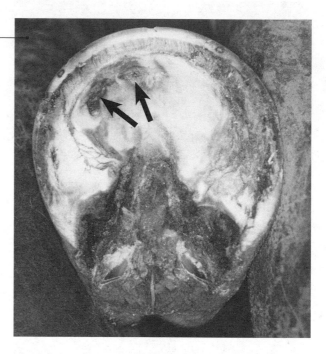

Sole Abscess

A sole bruise that becomes infected is an abscess. It is very painful and will cause acute lameness. With proper treatment, a sole abscess will usually heal in a week or two. However, if the infection spreads to the coffin bone, it could turn into a life-threatening situation.

SEEDY TOE AND WHITE LINE DISEASE

Seedy toe is a stretching or separating of the white line (junction of the sensitive and insensitive laminae). When a horse has seedy toe, his white line looks like a dry, fibrous cross-section of a grapefruit. It is a common result of founder (see page 128) and can also be caused by LT/LH and by prolonged exposure to moisture. Seedy toe opens the white line to invasion from dirt, moisture, and harmful organisms that cause thrush and white line disease.

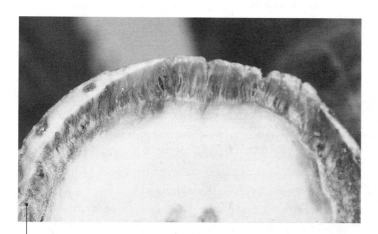

Open to Invasion

A stretched and separated white line is very porous, especially if the horse is barefoot. But even if he is shod, dirt and bacteria can be forced into the open spaces every time he takes a step.

White line disease (WLD) is an invasion of the white line by varieties of bacteria, fungus, and yeast that feed on the soft inner hoof horn. It can destroy the hoof laminae from the ground to the coronary band, leaving behind a hollow space that's sometimes filled with thrush or a white cheesy material. Loss of the laminae means loss of support and often results in rotation of the coffin bone, as with laminitis.

WLD seems to occur more frequently in hot, humid climates than in dry, cool areas. Symptoms of this disease are similar to those of laminitis: lameness; hoof heat; slow hoof growth; the development of a flat, sensitive sole; and sensitivity to nailing.

One method of treating mild cases of WLD involves either a farrier or the vet cleaning out as much of the affected hoof tissue as possible and then flushing and packing the hollow space with an antiseptic. A shoe is applied to protect the space and to keep the medication in place. The application of a CVP gasket pad (see Resource Guide and page 66) can aid in the recovery of hooves with WLD. The hooves must be kept in a dry environment and the shoes reset regularly, with the hoof treatment repeated each time.

In a severe case of WLD, the veterinarian may find it necessary to remove sections of the undermined hoof wall to properly treat the diseased area.

CLUBFOOT

A clubfoot is characterized by a hoof that is steeper than normal with a short toe and a long heel. Sometimes a steep hoof causes the horse no movement problems or discomfort. In these cases, it is usually better to leave the hoof alone rather than try to make it match the other hoof or trim it to look "normal."

Another type of clubfoot affects a hoof that has been non–weight bearing for a period of time, because of an injury, for example. The foot basically shrinks up and grows a long heel because it is not bearing weight. This is usually a temporary condition that will return to normal with proper trimming and sufficient exercise.

A third, more serious type of clubfoot is caused by a contraction of the flexor muscle-tendon unit that attaches to the coffin bone (tendons themselves don't contract). This can affect one or both front feet. It's not always clear why this happens, but as the muscle tightens, the tendon pulls the heel of the hoof off the ground and the heel grows very long. The horse's weight is shifted onto the toe, which causes excessive wear and dishing of the toe. Trying to forcibly lower the heels by trimming them short is rarely effective.

Successful approaches involve giving support to the heels and/or frog by means of an elevated heel shoe, boot, or pad so that the heels can bear weight. These methods take some weight off the toe and lessen the constant strain on the deep flexor muscle-tendon unit. It may allow the muscle to relax enough for the hoof to be gradually lowered to a more normal angle over a period of weeks.

In some cases, the heels might never be lowered to a normal angle, but the horse will still be comfortable and able to move without difficulty.

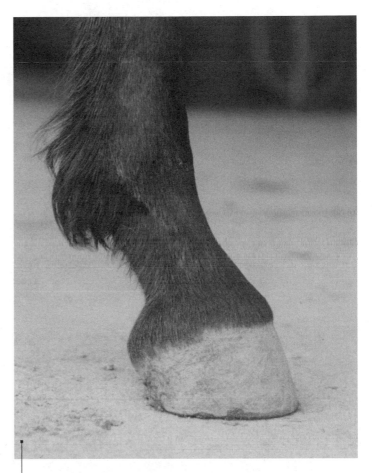

Steep Foal Hooves Are Often Normal

Many foals have naturally steep hoof angles — as high as 70 degrees. Usually, the steep hoof angle gradually comes down into the normal adult range within 3 to 16 months. In some cases this requires corrective trimming. If diagnosed and treated early, foals with clubfeet and accompanying contracted tendons have a fair chance to perform unencumbered as adults.

Advances in glue-on shoe technology allow corrective shoes to be applied to foals at a few weeks of age. However, it is difficult to predict which foals will respond to treatment. Yearlings who have had extensive corrective trimming and shoeing to correct clubfeet may look normal, but X-rays often show changes in the coffin bone that indicate a poor chance for the young horse to perform as an athlete.

OFF

Around horses, the word "off" has many meanings. The *off* side refers to the right side of a horse. A horse that's not feeling well might lose his appetite and go *off* his feed. And when a horse is traveling abnormally but is not quite lame, he is said to be *off*.

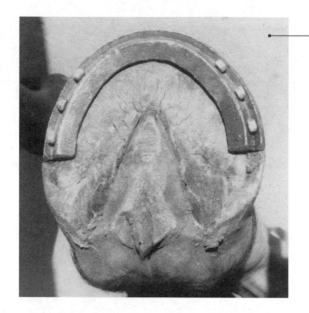

Tip Shoe Prevents Toe Wear

Mild clubfoot is sometimes caused by excessive wear of the bare toe from pawing or toe dragging or a poor-quality hoof wall. This can often be controlled by the application of a **half shoe,** also called a **tip shoe.** Usually made from the toe portion of a light shoe such as a training plate, the half shoe protects the toe of the hoof and leaves the heels bare to wear down in a normal fashion. The ends of the half shoe are tapered and/or set into the hoof, so there is not an abrupt step where the shoe ends and the quarters of the hoof begin. A benefit of the half shoe is that it cannot be stepped on and pulled off!

RICHARD'S CASE NOTES

Clubfoot

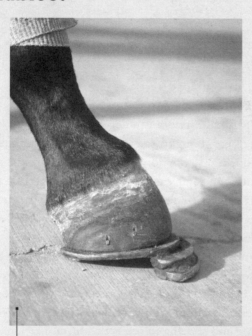

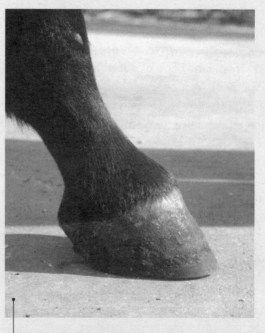

Elevated Toe Shoe Following Surgery

The clubfoot on this young horse was very severe and persisted despite months of treatment. The final option was a **tenotomy** — surgery to cut the tendon so the heel could relax. After surgery, a shoe with an elevated toe was applied to keep the hoof and pastern in a normal alignment while the tendon healed.

Back to Normal

The filly graduated in a few weeks from the elevated-toe shoe to a tip shoe (as pictured above), and now, several months later, her feet appear normal. Although she will probably never be a top athlete, she is moving so well on pasture that you'd never suspect she once had severe clubfoot.

NAVICULAR SYNDROME

Navicular syndrome is lameness in the front feet that involves the navicular bone itself and/or parts of the foot associated with it. One of the main causes of navicular syndrome is a long toe/low heel hoof configuration. This condition puts extreme and constant pressure on the navicular bone, even when the horse is standing still. The result is inflammation and pain. A navicular horse is sometimes said to be "heel sore."

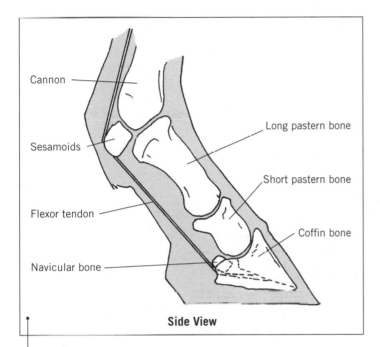

Cannon
Sesamoids
Flexor tendon
Navicular bone
Long pastern bone
Short pastern bone
Coffin bone

Side View

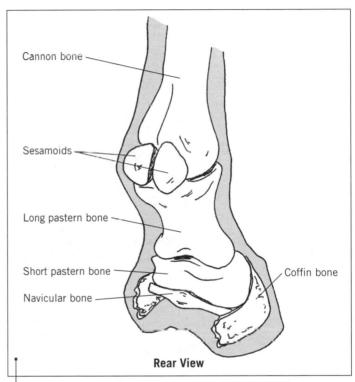

Cannon bone
Sesamoids
Long pastern bone
Short pastern bone
Navicular bone
Coffin bone

Rear View

A Pulley that Supports the Horse
The flexor tendon puts a tremendous amount of stress on the small navicular bone. It presses against the bone and slides up and down over it to support the weight of the horse and to lift the hoof as he moves forward.

Navicular Bone
The navicular bone, which is only about 2 inches (5 cm) long and less than ½ inch (1.3 cm) in diameter, is located at the back and bottom of the foot between the wings of the coffin bone.

SYMPTOMS OF NAVICULAR SYNDROME

If your horse demonstrates the following symptoms, he may be suffering from navicular syndrome:

- Progressive lameness involving one or both forelimbs
- A stiff, shuffling gait with a short, choppy stride
- Sensitivity to hoof testers when the central third of the frog is compressed
- A positive response to nerve blocking (low palmar digital nerve block)
- One hoof smaller and more upright than the other (if only one foot is affected)

- Contracted heels in one or both feet
- Hooves landing toe first when walking or trotting
- Stumbling
- Lameness of the inside foot when the horse is circled
- Increased lameness after a sharp turn
- Resting or pointing of the most severely affected foot to take weight off it or alternate pointing of both feet

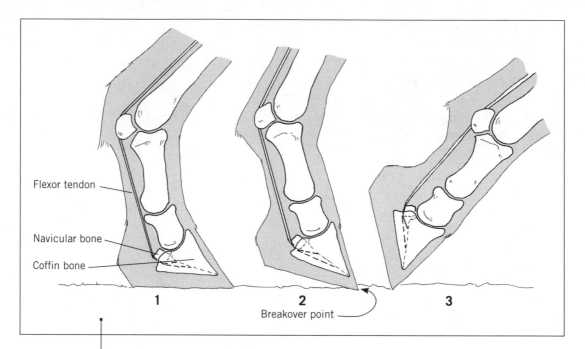

Flexor tendon

Navicular bone

Coffin bone

1   2   3

Breakover point

Breakover and the Navicular Bone

The hoof is like a lever with the toe as the pivot point. **Breakover** is the action of the hoof as it pivots over the toe to lift and move the leg forward.

1. Lifting force comes from the flexor tendon. As it pulls on the coffin bone to move the foot, the tendon presses on the navicular bone.

2. The longer the toe of the hoof, the more force it takes to lift the weight of the horse over the breakover point at the toe and the more pressure is put on the navicular bone.

3. As the foot leaves the ground, pressure on the navicular bone is reduced until the foot lands again.

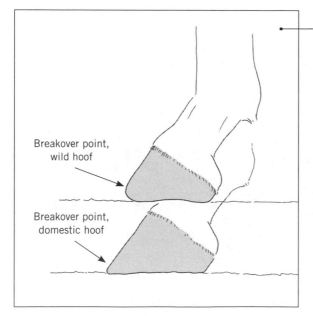

Breakover point, wild hoof

Breakover point, domestic hoof

Breakover of Wild and Domestic Horses

A wild horse's hoof typically has a short rounded toe, which puts the breakover point well under the foot. However, barefoot and shod domestic horses often have a longer toe that puts the breakover point much farther forward than that of a wild horse's hoof. This longer toe is the cause of many hoof problems.

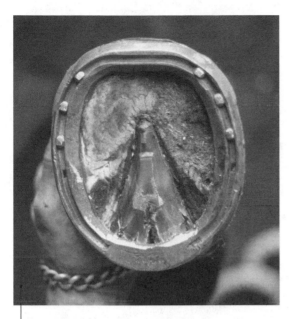

Navicular Prescription: Squared Toe Egg Bar

A simple and often effective treatment for navicular syndrome entails balancing the feet and applying an egg bar shoe with a rocker or a square toe, as shown here. Either shoe will move the pivot point of the hoof back under the foot (see page 63). This makes breakover less stressful and reduces pressure on the navicular bone.

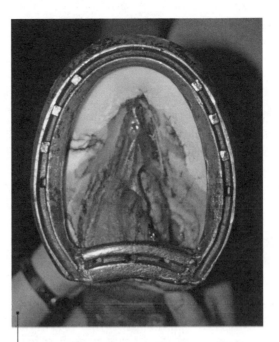

Straight Bar Shoe Protects Navicular Area

Horses suffering heel soreness from navicular syndrome or another cause are sensitive to pressure and concussion to the frog and heel area. A straight bar shoe like the one shown here can protect the back of the hoof area from ground contact while also making the horse more comfortable.

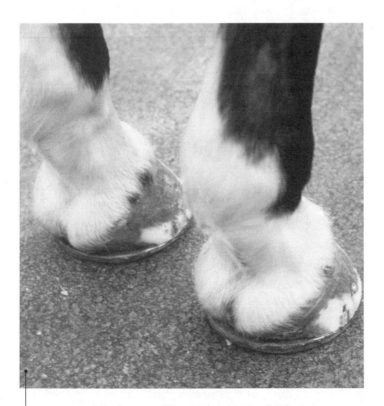

Egg Bar Shoe Provides Needed Heel Support

The egg bar shoe extends rearward to give the leg a larger base of support and keep the heels of the hoof from sinking down into soft footing.

Richard says . . .

EGG BARS TO THE RESCUE

Many horses I see that are diagnosed with navicular syndrome also have low and/or underrun heels. A British vet I worked with used to say, "The feet are crying out for egg bar shoes." Some horses are more comfortable and have shown dramatic improvement in comfort and movement immediately after the hooves were balanced and egg bar shoes applied. Others show more gradual improvement over days or weeks.

Until recently, a farrier had to make his egg bars. Today there is a good selection of factory-made egg bar shoes available.

LAMINITIS

Laminitis is a painful inflammation of the sensitive laminae inside the hoof. It is the second leading cause of death in horses (after colic). When laminae are damaged and the coffin bone tears loose from the hoof and sinks or rotates downward, it is called **founder**.

Laminitis most often affects the front feet but can affect any or all of the feet. For example, when the famous racehorse Barbaro broke his right hind leg and was unable to stand on it, his left hind foot soon developed laminitis from having to constantly bear the extra weight.

It is likely that many horses experience mild laminitis, with accompanying slight lameness, and recover without being diagnosed.

Horses that suffer significant hoof damage from laminitis (founder), resulting in weeks or months of unsoundness, are unlikely to ever return to their maximum level of performance, although some horses may become sound enough for light turnout and riding.

Horses that have foundered have been known to founder again. That's because permanent damage can occur in the foot and increase the risk of laminitis. Mares who have foundered may not be able to bear the additional weight and stress of a pregnancy without foundering again.

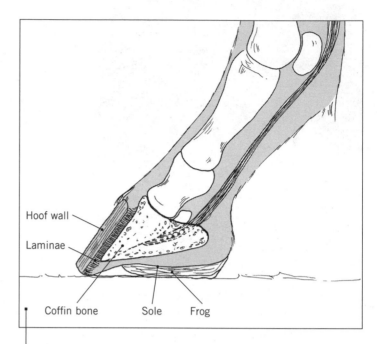

Laminae Connect Hoof Wall to Coffin Bone

The sensitive laminae on the coffin bone interlock with insensitive laminae on the inside of the hoof capsule to "laminate" the coffin bone to the hoof. The coffin bone is primarily suspended from the laminae and is somewhat supported by the sole and frog. In a healthy hoof, the front of the coffin bone is parallel to the front of the hoof wall and the laminae are an even thickness from the coronary band to the ground. (See page 3.)

RICHARD'S CASE NOTES

Sometimes We Win

I first saw Katie's 17-year-old Arabian gelding, Sundog, one September at the Vet Hospital. Sundog had turned up lame the day before and the exam confirmed laminitis in both fronts; the hinds were unaffected. I made a pair of heart bar shoes and applied them to Sundog's fronts. Katie trailered him home to a clean, bedded stall. I checked him the following week and found his comfort level had improved considerably. Every two weeks, I looked in on Sundog. I reset the shoes seven weeks after they were first applied and trimmed the bare hinds. Thereafter, I reset the shoes every five to six weeks.

At eight months: Sundog was enjoying limited turnout exercise in a small pen and showed little sign of lameness. He graduated from heart bar shoes to plain shoes. I used full pads and medicated hoof packing to protect the sole (which was still thin and tender) and to keep the damaged white line from becoming infected.

At 14 months: The soles had grown sufficient thickness to not need full pads. I switched to tube rim pads to prevent uncomfortable snowballing during the upcoming snowy season. Sundog was sound, and Katie used him for short rides.

At 24 months: Sundog remained sound. There was still some separation of the white line in places on both front hooves. I cleaned and packed those hollow areas with medication at each shoeing. With continued good management and regular hoof care Katie and Sundog enjoyed many more years together.

In the diagram labels: Hoof wall, Laminae, Coffin bone, Sole, Frog

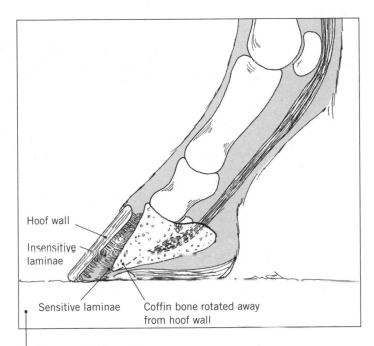

Separated Laminae

Laminitis is inflammation of the laminae that bind the hoof wall to the coffin bone. When the sensitive laminae are damaged or destroyed, they lose their grip on the insensitive laminae. Founder occurs when the weight of the horse and the pull of the deep flexor tendon cause the coffin bone to rotate and/or sink within the hoof capsule.

Hoof wall
Insensitive laminae
Sensitive laminae
Coffin bone rotated away from hoof wall

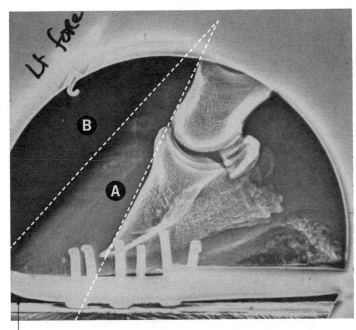

A Look Inside

X-rays let your veterinarian and farrier see the position of the coffin bone in the hoof capsule. You can see above that the coffin bone (**A**) has rotated so it is no longer parallel to the front of the hoof wall (**B**) as it should be. Venograms, which show blood flow in the foot, are another tool veterinarians and farriers can use at the onset of laminitis to determine damage affecting the blood flow of the foot and how best to direct treatment.

RICHARD'S CASE NOTES

Sometimes We Lose

Referred by a veterinarian, I began working on Tally, an overweight 16-year-old Quarter Horse mare. Her owner, Lisa, informed me that Tally foundered on the fronts four years ago and every spring since. She'd be lame for a few weeks, like now, but then get better. For Tally, the vet and I agreed, there should be no pasture, no grain, limited exercise, and only grass hay. I trimmed Tally's long toes and shod her with egg bar shoes and frog support pads.

At two weeks: Lisa said Tally was improving but "wants to get out of her pen and eat grass." Permission denied.

At five weeks: At the scheduled reset time, Tally's hooves had barely grown, but she had lost some weight. I pulled the shoes, checked the soles (they looked fine), replaced the hoof packing, and reset the shoes using the same nail holes.

At six weeks: Lisa called saying Tally had lost a shoe. "Did you find it in her pen?" I asked.

"No, it must be out in the pasture . . . " Lisa said.

The grazing was bad enough but a sudden thunderstorm scared Tally into a long gallop that made her dead lame on both fronts. I suggested Lisa call her vet, who sent the horse straight to the hospital.

Tally was at the hospital for two weeks, treated by the best vets in the region, consulting with the best vets in the country. After Tally went home I provided the hoof care (sometimes weekly) they prescribed. But it was a losing battle.

At four months: Tally lay in her stall, getting up only with great difficulty. It was painfully apparent that she wasn't getting better. After untold heartache and tens of thousands of dollars for the best care available, Lisa made the decision to have Tally euthanized.

Causes of Laminitis

- Overeating of grain or pasture grasses
- Extra weight (overweight horses and mares in foal) puts constant excess stress on a horse's feet
- Inflammation of the gastrointestinal tract
- Cushing's disease, an abnormality of the pituitary gland that results in excessive cortisol, a natural steroid hormone
- Insulin resistance; prevents sugars from reaching the cells and causes a horse to store sugar as fat
- Trimming the hooves too short
- Seedy toe, when bacteria infect the laminae
- Penetrating hoof injuries
- Retention of the placenta during foaling
- Physical trauma to the feet, such as prolonged exercise on a hard surface
- Exposure to black walnut wood shavings
- Allergic reactions to certain plants or medications
- Large doses of corticosteroids
- A diet containing estrogens
- Prolonged weightbearing on one leg, such as when the opposite leg is non–weight bearing because of injury
- Other nonspecific forms of stress

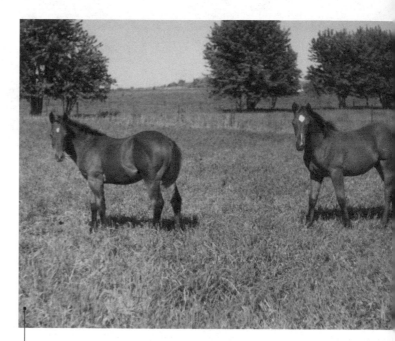

Limit Grazing

Overeating, especially of grain or pasture grasses that are high in sugar, is one of the main causes of laminitis. When a horse eats more than he can readily digest, the undigested feed ferments in the horse's gut and leads to an overabundance of undesirable bacteria that cause laminitis.

Because pasture sugar content changes with seasons, weather, temperature, and time of day, grazing should be carefully managed.

Grasses are highest in sugars:

- When plants are stressed by drought or frost
- When blooming or heading
- When cut very short by mowing or grazing
- When still green after freezing temperatures
- In the late afternoon
- On sunny days

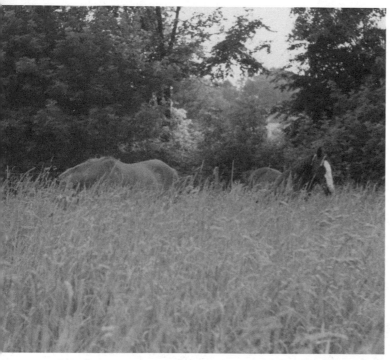

Tall mature grass is usually low in sugar and high in fiber so is safe for grazing.

Cherry says . . .

LIMIT SUGAR

The safest times to let your horse graze on pasture are early in the morning and on cloudy days, when sugar content is low. The safest grasses for your horse to eat are tall, mature grass and dead, brown winter grass; both are high in fiber and low in sugar.

Symptoms of Laminitis

Signs of laminitis will vary depending on the horse and on the severity of the disease. Because the sensitive laminae are trapped between the hard coffin bone and the rigid hoof wall, they have no room to expand when they become inflamed, and the pain can be excruciating.

Here are some signs to watch for:
- Increased digital pulse rate
- Increased temperature in the hoof and coronary band
- Swelling of the coronary band
- Continual lifting of the feet every few seconds
- Lameness, especially when the horse is walked or longed in a circle
- Extreme sensitivity to hoof testers over the sole in front of the frog (See photo page 138 of hoof testers in use.)
- Standing with the forelegs out in front and the hind legs up underneath
- Reluctance or refusal to walk
- Lying down for extended periods
- Trembling, anxiety, rapid respiration, and increased rectal temperature

(See photo page 138 of hoof testers in use.)

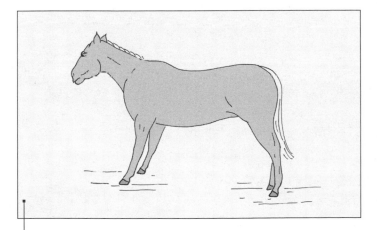

Laminitic Stance
A horse with laminitis in his front feet will typically assume the "saw horse" or "A-frame" stance, with the front legs stretched out to take weight off the toes and carry it on the heels. If the hind feet are affected, the horse will place them well underneath his body to shift weight to the heels.

See photo page 138

Cherry says . . .

KNOW NORMAL VITAL SIGNS

To know what normal vital signs are for your horse, check his pulse, respiration, and temperature twice a day for three days when he is healthy and at rest. Average the readings. Choose various times of day, but always conduct the checks when the horse is at rest, not when he has just been working or is excited. Write the averages down, and keep them with your horse's health records, where you can find them.

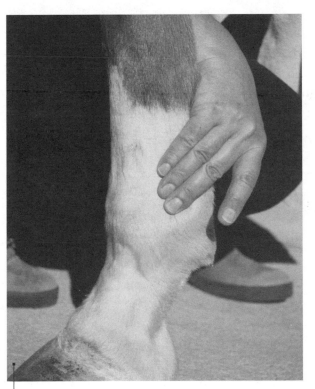

Checking a Horse's Pulse
You can easily check your horse's pulse on the maxillary artery, located on the inside of the jawbone, and on the digital artery, located on both the inside and outside of the horse's leg, just above the fetlock.

Press your fingertips lightly against an artery until you feel the horse's pulse. Count the beats for 60 seconds, or if your horse is restless, count for 15 seconds and then multiply by 4 to get the pulse rate per minute. The normal range is 30 to 40 beats per minute.

Treatment of Laminitis

Laminitis is a medical emergency that requires immediate diagnosis and treatment. If you have reason to suspect that your horse has laminitis, do not wait to see what happens. While you are waiting, his hooves could be dying inside, and he could founder. The sooner you, your veterinarian, and your farrier all leap into action, the better chance you'll have of preventing founder and sparing your horse unnecessary suffering.

Find the best professionals you can. If your veterinarian and farrier are unsure about treatment, don't hesitate to ask them to refer you to more experienced colleagues.

Immediate care can include:

- Anti-inflammatory drugs
- In the case of grain overload, passing a tube to the horse's gut and administering mineral oil to act as a laxative and to coat the intestinal lining to prevent absorption of toxins
- Soaking the affected feet (to the knees if possible) for long periods in circulating cold water
- Confining the horse to a sand stall
- Allowing the horse to lie down if he chooses, to keep weight off his feet

There is no one best treatment for all cases of laminitis. Current approaches that have worked on some horses and failed on others include:

- Raising the heels
- Lowering the heels
- Supporting only the frog and outer hoof wall
- Supporting all or part of the sole
- Shoeing
- Leaving the horse barefoot

Besides initial emergency care, a horse suffering from severe laminitis will need frequent farrier attention and periodic veterinary care for a year and maybe longer. Although experienced professionals can set the stage for a horse's recovery, the owner's long-term commitment to the treatment program is of paramount importance. Many cases will require daily treatment, specialized management, and close dietary supervision for the life of the horse. In spite of the most conscientious treatment by the best professionals and a committed owner, however, some horses with severe laminitis will fail to improve and will eventually need to be euthanized.

Cherry says . . .

WEIGH YOUR OPTIONS THOUGHTFULLY

I have often traveled with Richard and was there on a number of occasions when he worked on laminitic horses. I saw that dealing with laminitis requires emotional strength and a considerable investment of time and money. Many horses do not recover. A horse with serious laminitis suffers for months or years whether he recovers or not.

As a caring horse owner, look honestly at your motives and interest in your horse, and weigh them against the horse's comfort level and quality of life during and after treatment for laminitis. Then discuss euthanasia with your veterinarian at the outset of treatment and at various times along the way.

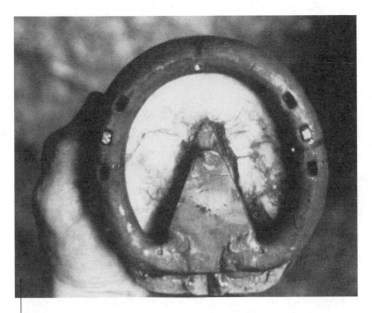

Heart Bar Shoe

Shoeing options for laminitis include the heart bar shoe and heart bar pad. The shoe or pad can be modified from a commercial product or be handmade and applied by an experienced farrier.

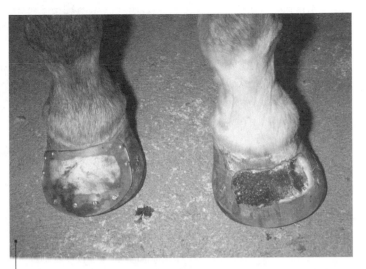

Window Resection

In some cases a section, or window, of hoof wall is removed (**resected**) at the front of a foundered hoof to keep dead, deformed laminae from interfering with new hoof growth. A removable plastic cover attached with screws (above, left) keeps the site clean and enables the application of medication.

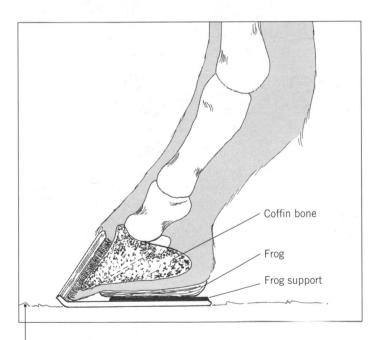

Coffin bone

Frog

Frog support

Frog Support

The heart bar shoe or pad is carefully designed and precisely applied to support a very specific area of the frog in order to prevent or minimize the rotation of the coffin bone within the hoof capsule. The farrier will need to see recent X-rays of the foot in order to place the frog support correctly.

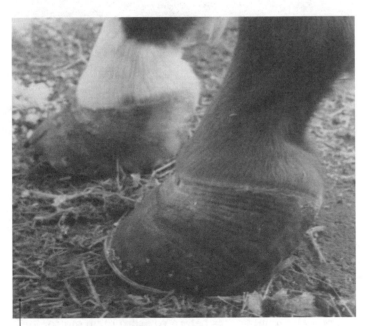

Founder Rings Show History

When a horse founders, the laminae holding the hoof to the coffin bone die and tear apart and the coffin bone rotates downward. Founder often damages blood vessels that feed the front portion of the hoof, so the heels grow faster than the toe, resulting in wavy growth rings. These "founder rings" are one of the most easily recognizable signs that a horse has foundered.

Preventing Laminitis

Laminitis has been likened to type II diabetes in humans, in part because some of the main symptoms of both diseases are detected in the feet. As with diabetes, one of the foremost preventive measures taken for laminitis entails carefully monitoring how much sugar the horse is ingesting.

The following guidelines are sensible for all horses but should be strictly observed if your horse tends to get fat or has had laminitis before:

- Avoid feeding your horse sweet treats like sugar cubes and carrots
- Minimize feeding grain, especially sweet feeds containing molasses, corn syrup, or other sweeteners (beet pulp and soy hulls are a safer source of calories)
- Avoid feeding hay that was cut in early growth stages or during times of stressful weather such as drought (hay that has started to seed generally has a lower sugar content)
- Have your hay tested for mineral and sugar content so you know what you are feeding your horse and what nutrients are lacking

- Feed a balanced diet, including mineral supplements if your hay tests show this is necessary
- Soak high-sugar or suspect hay for 60 minutes in cold water before feeding; this can reduce its sugar content by one-third
- Maintain your horse at a healthy weight

Other measures you can take to prevent laminitis:
- Have hooves trimmed regularly by a professional farrier
- Check paddocks, pens, and other places your horse spends time to ensure the ground is free of nails, wire, staples, screws, or other objects that could puncture his hoof (check local rental stores for long floor magnets that you can pull over the ground to find hidden hazards)
- Provide adequate exercise, by leading, active turnout (not grazing!), riding, longeing, driving, ponying, or other forms

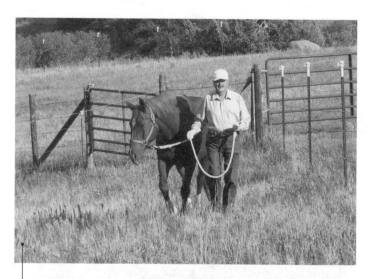

Limit Grazing, No Matter What Your Horse Thinks

Limit the time your horse is allowed to graze, especially if he's an "easy keeper." Introduce grazing on pasture gradually to all horses before you turn them out for longer periods. Some horses cannot safely be out on pasture full time.

For the first few days, allow your horse to graze on pasture for 15 minutes twice a day. After a few days let him graze for half an hour twice daily. Finally, give him one hour twice a day. If a horse shows the slightest sign of hoof soreness when you bring him in, cut back on or eliminate grazing time.

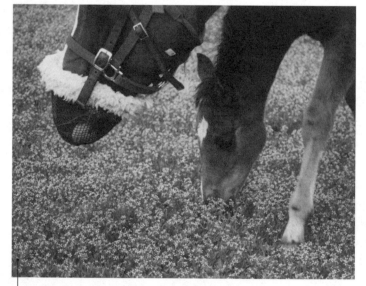

Grazing Muzzle

A well-fitted grazing muzzle can allow a horse to be turned out for exercise while limiting the amount of grass he can eat. Be sure to check the horse several times throughout the day to make sure the muzzle is still on and that he hasn't caught it on something. It's good insurance to use a breakaway halter if the muzzle attaches to a halter or to use a breakaway attachment on the muzzle so that if the muzzle does catch on a post or other object it will come off without injuring your horse.

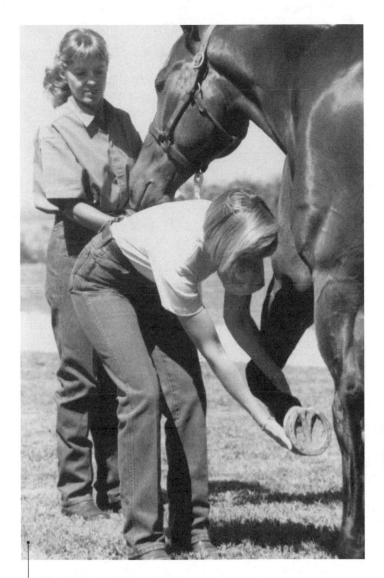

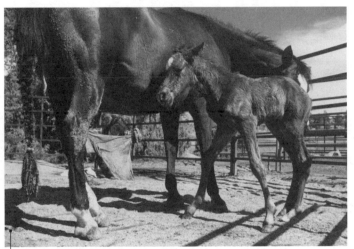

Cherry says . . .

BE A GOOD MIDWIFE

Foaling time is no time to be squeamish. It is your responsibility to verify that your mare expels the entire placenta. To see what you should be looking for check out a good foaling book, ask your vet, search the Internet, and talk with horse owner friends who've been around foaling. When in doubt, save the placenta in a clean bucket and ask your veterinarian to examine it as soon as possible.

Check Your Horse Daily

To prevent laminitis, check your horse daily for normal stance, movement, and comfort level. If you notice unusual behavior, take the horse's digital pulse and feel the hooves for elevated temperature.

Make Sure the Entire Placenta Is Expelled

Keep a close watch on your mare when she foals to make sure that the entire placenta is expelled soon after birthing. If even a small piece of placenta remains attached to the mare's uterus, it can result in a toxic buildup and laminitis.

Keep Grain Safe from Horses

One thing's for sure, horses don't know when to quit eating. Keep your grain and supplements in horseproof containers or in a locked feed room so that if a horse gets loose in the barn he will not be able to get at the feed, eat himself sick, and founder.

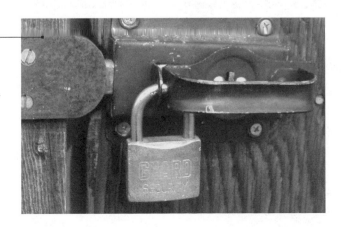

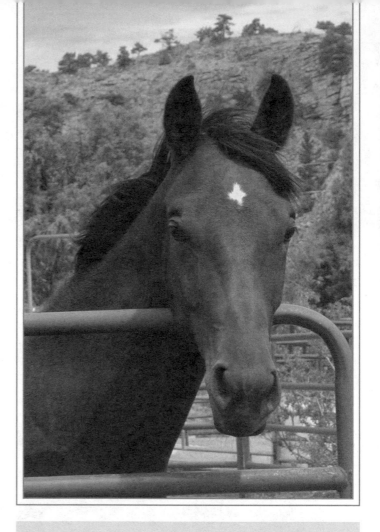

-13-
TEAMWORK

Your horse's comfort, soundness, and performance longevity are the result of a team effort. As the owner, you are team captain, and it is your responsibility to coordinate the efforts of all the other players: the horse, the veterinarian, and the farrier. If you board your horse, you'll also need to involve your barn manager. Similarly, if you use a trainer, he or she should be involved in any hoof care discussion.

The Silent Partner

Your horse is the reason the team exists, but he is also a silent partner. He has no say in who is on his team, let alone where he lives, how he eats, or what he does for a living. He is totally dependent on you to make wise decisions for him and to select the very best team members to attend to his hoof care.

Richard says . . .

KEEPING THE PEACE

Ideally, your veterinarian and farrier are both team players, but sometimes methods and egos collide. A veterinarian has earned his credentials through years of intense formal education and internship. A farrier, with or without formal hoof-care classes, has gathered invaluable experience from daily work on horses' feet. Each might have a different opinion on how to treat a given case and both might feel they are "right."

It is up to a horse's owner to be the team referee, diplomat, and judge, in order to get the best treatment for the horse. Confrontations can often be avoided by making sure that both the farrier and the vet are consulted and kept up-to-date on treatment plans and decisions made in their absence. When all attempts at diplomacy fail, it might be necessary to replace either your farrier or veterinarian for the benefit of the horse.

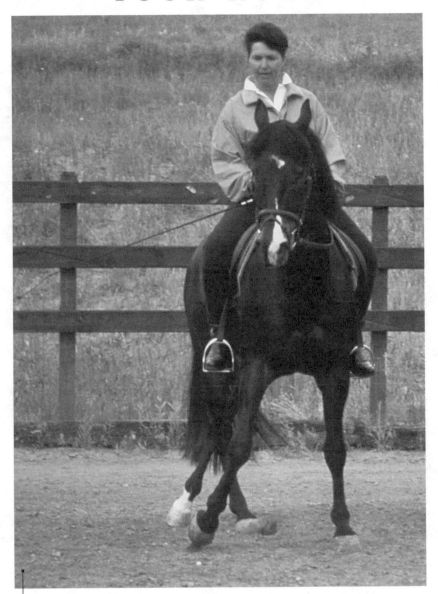

Team Captain

You are responsible for providing competent care and management of the horse, which includes plenty of exercise; healthy feed; adequate, clean housing; consistent veterinary and farrier care; regular grooming; and proper training. A rider should be closely tuned to her horse's movement to detect subtle changes that might indicate a problem. The owner should make sure the place the horse lives and his daily management routines are geared toward healthy hooves.

When you board your horse away from home or you hire someone to perform training and management duties at your barn, that person is essentially your horse's manager and handler. He or she is responsible daily for your horse's safety, diet, and comfort. But even when the care or training of a horse is entrusted to another person, it is still the owner's responsibility to see that things are done correctly and decisions are made in the best interest of the horse.

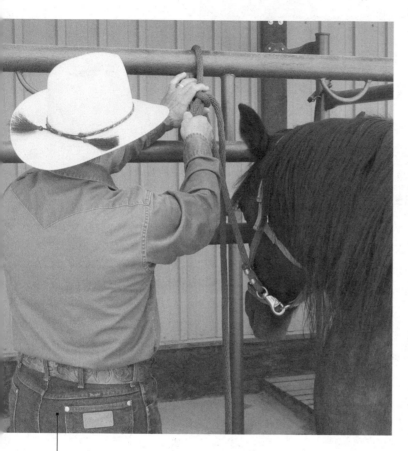

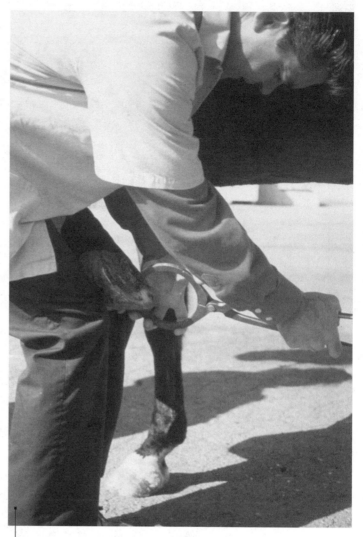

Good Manners Begin at Home

The owner is responsible for seeing that a horse is taught good ground manners so he is relaxed and comfortable with shoeing procedures and is safe to work around. A horse should learn to stand quietly when tied and allow a farrier or veterinarian to handle and work on his feet.

An Equine Vet Is Essential

Employ the services of a conscientious equine veterinarian who stays abreast of ongoing research, shoeing techniques, lameness diagnoses, and treatments. Encourage your veterinarian to interact with your farrier. They should both be involved in prepurchase evaluations and help you formulate a management program for your horse to ensure healthy feet. The combination of their knowledge and experience will benefit both you and your horse.

SCHEDULING A FARRIER VISIT

Scheduling conflicts and miscommunication are the most common obstacles to obtaining continuous farrier service. To ensure that you and your farrier can stay on schedule for your horse's sake, find out your farrier's preference for handling appointments. Does he schedule appointments seven weeks in advance? If so, do you have to confirm the appointment the day before, or do you both just show up? Does the farrier require you or someone else to be present when he is working? What happens if one of you misses the appointment?

Some farriers prefer clients to call close to the time of shoeing to set a date for an appointment. If so, know when you should call. Does he want to pencil you in three weeks ahead or the day before? You should have an idea of how long after you call him you can expect to get an appointment.

When making the appointment, have an accurate list of your trimming and shoeing needs available to refer to. If these change before your appointment, have the courtesy to call your farrier so he can adjust his schedule accordingly. Be sure to mention your horse's special problems or needs so your shoer can bring necessary supplies. Although some farriers' trucks are veritable stores, filled with an assortment of shoes, pads, nails, and accessories, other farriers like to travel light. If your horse has unusually large or small feet, needs studs, polo shoes, sliders, or snow pads, or requires quarter-crack repair, let your farrier know so he can arrived prepared.

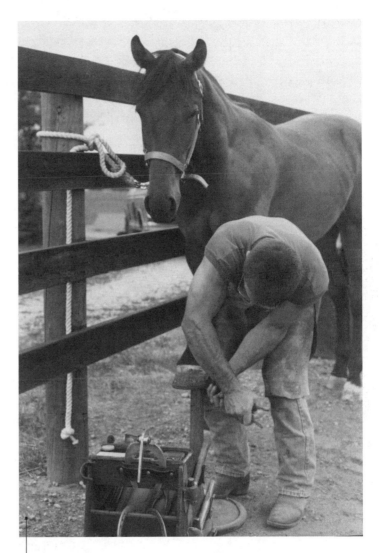

Your Farrier

The farrier's primary role is to trim and shoe the horse, with the objective of keeping the feet balanced and protecting them from injury. The farrier's goals should be, first, long-term soundness and, second, optimal performance. Depending on the extent of your farrier's experience, he may also be able to assist your veterinarian in the treatment of various hoof and limb problems. Ask your farrier to participate in prepurchase examinations, as his specialized hoof experience might allow him to spot hoof problems or tendencies missed by even top-notch veterinarians.

Richard says . . .

KEEP COMMUNICATION CLEAR

To keep my shoeing business running smoothly, every one of my clients receives a four-page brochure. This handout contains my basic shoeing prices, lost shoe charges, cost of modifications such as clips and pads, and my mileage rate. There are also two lists. One describes what duties I perform and what procedures I will not do. The other list outlines what I expect from the horse owner. I've found that having these things in writing answers important questions and prevents misunderstandings.

KEEPING A GOOD FARRIER

Discuss payment arrangements with your farrier. Some farriers use a monthly billing system, especially with larger barns or clients with a lot of horses. Most, however, require payment at the time of service. If you won't be there in person, arrange to leave a check or cash; prompt payment will help ensure continued farrier service.

All horses that are scheduled for work should be readily available when your farrier arrives. They can be tied or cross-tied in the barn or in nearby stalls or small pens conveniently located near the working area.

To enable your farrier to do his very best work, provide him with a proper shoeing area and well-mannered horses. If your horses are muddy, be sure to clean them, especially the parts the farrier will rub up against or handle — their shoulders, hindquarters, and legs. Also, scrape and then wipe the mud off the hooves rather than hosing them off. Clean, dry hooves are much safer and more pleasant for the farrier to work on than slippery, wet hooves.

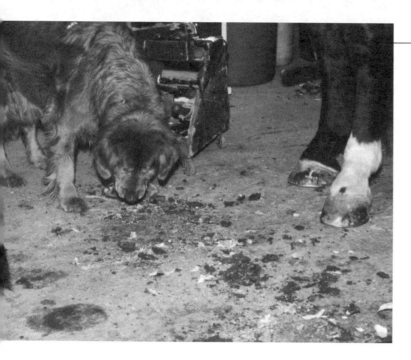

Dogs and Kids

Dogs love to chew hoof trimmings, but they can be seriously injured if they swallow old hoof packing, medicated trimmings, or nails. And even if a dog and horse are used to one another, a dog can get underfoot, distract the farrier, and cause an accident. The more the farrier is allowed to concentrate on his work without interruptions, the better the shoeing job, and the safer it will be for everyone. As much as your dog might want to be part of the team, it is best for the safety of all involved if his participation as part of the cleanup crew comes after the farrier or vet have completed their jobs and left and after you have picked up any harmful leavings.

The same goes for children. It is a learning experience for youngsters to become familiar with your vet and farrier and their roles in the care of your horse. However, they should be encouraged to ask questions when the time is right, such as during a break or after the work is done. In the interest of safety and to allow your professionals to do their best work, children and pets should not be allowed to distract or interfere with your farrier and vet while they are working on your horse.

One of the best ways to keep a good farrier is to be genuinely interested in the health of your horse's hooves. Be a conscientious manager and rider, and learn all you can about hoof care and shoeing. The more knowledgeable you are, the better able you will be to converse with your farrier about any hoof condition that arises. Stay informed by reading specialized books and articles related to shoeing.

The care of your horse's hooves is a team effort. Take the time to find a really interested, skilled farrier, then treat him like the professional he is, and you will likely be able to retain his good services.

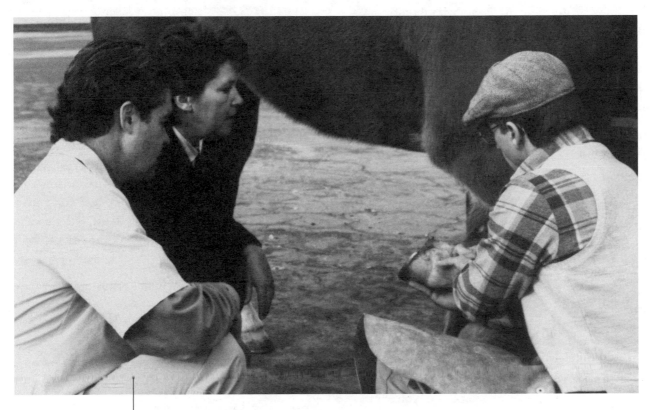

The Team
The combined interest and efforts of the owner, the vet, and the farrier, along with the cooperation of the horse, can ensure that he will remain sound, comfortable, and active throughout his lifetime.

Cherry says . . .

TREAT YOUR FARRIER WELL

Richard was a full-time farrier for 17 years, and I often rode with him for the day because he's great company! I also tagged along so I could take photos for our archives and meet the interesting people and horses in Richard's appointment book. These road trips gave me a bird's-eye view of the vast array of facilities, management, and manners (both human and equine). Horseshoeing is hard work! I really appreciate the great job he does on my horses, so I try to make things as comfortable and safe as I can for him.

FARRIER VISIT DOS AND DON'TS

DO offer to hold your horses rather than tie them if it is their first time for trimming or shoeing, but . . .

DON'T feel offended if your offer is rejected. Your farrier may prefer to work alone, with the horse tied.

DO have plenty of fly repellent on hand, but . . .

DON'T wait until your farrier's visit to acquaint your horse with a spray bottle, and . . .

DON'T spray the horse while your farrier is working under him.

DO introduce your dogs to your farrier, but . . .

DON'T let your dogs roam loose where the farrier is working.

DO tell your horseshoer the name, age, and use of each horse, but . . .

DON'T tell him about the last clinic you attended, about each trophy your horse has won, or the first time he saw a llama! You shouldn't expect your farrier to really listen or to carry on a conversation. He is there for one reason — to provide a professional service that allows you to participate in your favorite horse activities. The less attention he gives you, the more he can give to the work you are paying for.

DO pay attention to your horse's behavior, but . . .

DON'T take your nervous horse for a calming hike down the gravel driveway on freshly trimmed feet while the farrier is shaping his shoe.

DO discuss stable management and hoof care with your farrier. Ask him about the symptoms of problems he may see in your horse's feet, and listen to his recommendations to remedy them, but . . .

DON'T expect miracles from your farrier. If you bought a horse that had been neglected for two years, or if you have a horse with crooked legs, or if you board at a stable with muddy pens, don't think that your farrier has a magic rasp that can cure cracks, founder, conformation flaws, and thrush. You must work together toward gradual, permanent results.

DO have your payment in full ready for the farrier before he leaves, and . . .

DON'T make him ask.

DO offer him a place to wash up and a glass of water, and . . .

DON'T forget to write down the date and time of your next appointment.

REWARDS

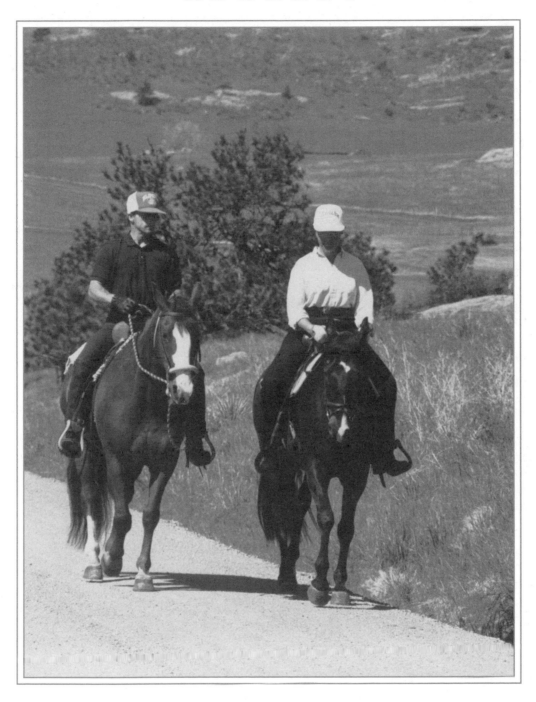

GLOSSARY

abscess. Infection in the foot that results from a hole or crack in the horny sole that permits the entry of contaminants; can also result from a bruise; pressure buildup causes extreme pain and lameness. Sometimes referred to as gravel.

AFA. American Farrier's Association; U.S.-based farrier organization founded in 1971.

anterior. On or toward the front.

anvil. Large block of steel with a hardened top surface on which metal (such as a horseshoe) is shaped using a hammer.

artery. Blood vessel that carries blood from the heart to the tissues.

axis. Line through the center of a body or body part.

balance, hoof. When the horse's weight is distributed equally over the hoof; see *DP balance* and *ML balance*.

bar shoe. Horseshoe that is connected at the heels; used to add support, apply pressure, prevent pressure, or stabilize the shoe or hoof.

bar stock. Metal bar from which horseshoes are forged.

bilateral. On both sides.

biotin. B-complex vitamin essential for health of hooves and hair; manufactured in the horse's gut; often included in horse-feed supplements.

blacksmith. Person who forges items from steel.

blowout. Horizontal crack in the hoof wall caused either by an injury to the coronary band or by a blow to the hoof wall.

borium. Tungsten carbide chips in a steel or brass matrix; applied to the ground surface of a horseshoe for traction or to increase wear.

branch. One-half of a horseshoe, from the toe to the heel.

breakover. Movement of a hoof from the time it begins to pivot over the toe until it leaves the ground.

bruise. Injury to the skin or sensitive tissue from a blow or collision that ruptures blood vessels but does not break the skin.

bulbs. Area at the back of the foot where the frog and hoof wall merge with the skin.

BWFA. Brotherhood of Working Farriers Association; U.S.-based farrier organization founded in 1989.

calk. Projection on the ground surface of a horseshoe used to increase traction, alter movement, or adjust stance. Also called caulk, calkin, cork, or sticker.

capsule. See *hoof capsule*.

caulk. See *calk*.

clinch. End of a horseshoe nail that is folded over to hold the horseshoe on the hoof; the part of a horseshoe nail visible on the outside of a shod horse's hoof; also called a clench.

clincher. Tool used for bending the end of a horseshoe nail over to form a clinch.

clip. Metal extension on the outside edge of a horseshoe that lies flat against the hoof or is burned into the hoof; used to help hold the shoe on or to stabilize the hoof.

close nail. Horseshoe nail driven into the hoof wall that puts pressure on the sensitive inner structures without actually piercing them.

clubfoot. Hoof imbalance, usually on one or both fronts, caused by an extremely upright hoof with a short toe and long heel.

coffin bone. Hoof-shaped bone at the end of the leg, located within the hoof capsule; also referred to as pedal bone, distal phalanx, distal phalange, third phalanx, PIII, P-3, and os pedis.

cold shoeing. Method of horseshoeing in which the shoe is not heated in a forge but is shaped and applied cold.

conformation. Inherited physical structure of a horse.

contracted heels. Heels of a hoof that are abnormally close together.

corium. Blood-rich tissue that lines the inside of the hoof and nourishes the parts of the foot.

corn. Bruise or abscess that occurs at the seat of corn, where the hoof wall curves to join the bars.

coronary band. Strip of tissue that produces most of the hoof wall; it runs around the top of the hoof just below the hairline. Also called the coronet.

coronet. See *coronary band*.

corrective trimming and shoeing. Trimming and shoeing with the purpose of altering a horse's stance or stride.

cow hocks. Hocks that are closer together than the hind feet.

crack. Separation or break in the surface of the hoof wall. Vertical cracks are referred to by their location, such as toe cracks, quarter cracks, and heel cracks. Cracks that originate at the coronary band are called sand cracks or coronary cracks, while those that start at the ground surface are called grass cracks. Surface cracks or superficial cracks are tiny fissures that cover varying portions of the hoof wall. A horizontal crack is a *blowout*.

crease. Groove in the ground surface of a horseshoe to provide a seat for the nail heads and to provide traction.

crease nail puller. Long-handled tool with narrow pointed jaws designed to grip the head of a horseshoe nail and pull it from the shoe.

deep digital flexor tendon (DDFT). Tendon that runs down the back of the leg, over the navicular bone, and connects to the bottom of the coffin bone.

degree pad. See *wedge pad*.

dish. Dip (concavity) in the front surface of the hoof wall.

distal. Away from the center, or torso; opposite of proximal.

dorsal. Front surface of a hoof and leg; or when referring to the entire horse, the spine, or the centerline of the back.

DP balance (dorsal palmar/plantar). Refers to the alignment of the hoof angle and the pastern angle, when viewed from the side; ideally, an imaginary line through the center of the *pastern (axis)* is parallel with the front of the hoof wall.

dropped sole. Sole that protrudes downward and has become convex rather than concave.

egg bar. Horseshoe that is connected at the heels and is oval shaped, like an egg; used to support weak hooves and legs and as a preventive measure on sound limbs.

expansion. Increase in hoof width at the heels when the foot bears weight; increase in circumference bottom of the hoof as it grows

longer; excess horseshoe width at the heels purposely fitted to accommodate hoof growth.

extended heel shoe. Horseshoe with heels that are longer than normal.

farrier. Professional horseshoer.

feral. Animal that runs free and that is or was domesticated or has ancestors that were domesticated.

flare. Dip (concavity) in the surface of the hoof wall, usually at the sides; a flare at the toe is called a dish.

float. To cut away a portion of the hoof wall at the heels so the heel does not bear weight on the horseshoe.

foot. Hoof and its internal structures, which include bones, the sensitive structures, the insensitive structures, and the elastic structures.

foot flight. The path a foot takes as it moves through the air from the time it leaves the ground until it lands.

forehand. The portion of the horse ahead of the heart girth; includes the front legs and shoulder.

forge. To make or alter an item from heated metal using a hammer and anvil; furnace usually fueled by coal or propane and used to heat metal.

forging. When the toe of a hind hoof or shoe strikes the sole or shoe of a front hoof; similar to, but not as extreme as, overreaching.

founder. Result of laminitis, where the coffin bone rotates or sinks within the hoof capsule.

frog. V-shaped rubbery tissue on the bottom of the hoof.

full pad. Pad inserted between hoof and shoe that covers the entire sole and frog.

full-support shoe. Combination of an egg bar and a heart bar shoe.

gravel. See *abscess*.

Guild of Professional Farriers (GPF). U.S.-based farrier organization founded in 1996.

hoof. Hard external foot below the coronary band, including the hoof wall, sole, and frog.

hoof angle. Relationship between the front (dorsal) wall of the hoof and the ground. The hoof angle is considered correct when the hoof and pastern are in alignment: that is, the front surface of the hoof is parallel to an imaginary line through the center of the long pastern bone.

hoof boot. Hoof covering made of synthetic materials such as rubber and plastic that is used instead of horseshoes when riding, to protect a hoof that loses a shoe or that is injured, and to soak an injured hoof for treatment.

hoof capsule. Hard outer shell of the hoof that encases the sensitive structures.

hoof dressing. Paste or cream applied to the hoof for the purpose of improving hoof quality.

hoof gauge. Tool for measuring hoof angle.

hoof horn. Tough, insensitive fibers that make up the hoof wall and sole.

hoof rings. Lines or ridges around the circumference of the hoof wall; can be caused by changes in diet, environment, season, or by illness; very pronounced hoof rings could indicate the horse has been foundered. Also called growth rings and fever rings.

hoof sealer. Liquid or gel applied to the hoof wall to help maintain moisture balance by minimizing the amount of moisture the hoof absorbs from the environment and the amount that evaporates from within the hoof.

hoof tester. Device used to apply local pressure to various spots on the hoof to locate sources of pain and sensitivity.

horn. See *hoof horn*.

horseshoe. Device attached to the bottom of the hoof to protect it from wear and damage, provide support, and add or remove traction; commonly made of steel, aluminum, or plastic; usually applied using nails but sometimes glued.

hot fitting. Pressing a hot shoe against the bottom of the hoof; scorched spots on the hoof then indicate high areas that need to be rasped away for a proper fit; if the shoe is hot enough, it will melt the hoof horn and result in a perfect fit between the shoe and the hoof.

hot nail. Horseshoe nail that is driven into the sensitive structures of the hoof.

hot shoeing. Method of horseshoeing in which the shoe is heated to be shaped; can be used with keg shoes or handmade shoes; may or may not involve hot fitting.

interfering. When a horse hits the inside of a leg or foot with the opposite hoof.

keg shoe. Factory-made shoe.

keratin. Tough protein component in horn, hair, skin, and hooves.

knock-kneed. Conformation where the knees bend inward and are closer together than the feet.

lameness. Pain or physical defect that interferes with normal movement; evidenced by varying degrees of limping.

laminae. The tissues that attach the hoof wall to the coffin bone. The inner, sensitive laminae attach to the coffin bone, and the outer, insensitive or horny laminae attach to the inside surface of the hoof wall.

laminitis. Acute inflammation of the sensitive laminae in the hoof; can be caused by a wide variety of factors, including overeating of grain or pasture grasses, trauma, and foaling complications. The chronic form of the condition is often referred to as founder.

limb. Entire equine appendage, from the scapula or hip down.

long toe/low heel (LT/LH). Hoof imbalance where the toe is abnormally long in relation to the length of the heels; can result in excess flexor tendon stress and cause heel soreness, cracks, contracted heels, and development of navicular syndrome.

ML balance (medio-lateral). Relationship between the medial (inside) wall of the hoof and the lateral (outside) wall of the hoof, and the position and weight bearing of the hoof under the leg.

natural collection. Balanced movement.

natural trimming. Method of trimming that models the shape of feral horse hooves.

navicular bone. Small bone located between the wings of the coffin bone; acts like a pulley for the flexor tendon, which runs over it. Also called the distal sesamoid bone.

navicular syndrome. Chronic lameness involving the navicular bone and associated structures, almost exclusively affecting the forelimbs.

off. Slightly lame.

overreaching. Gait defect where the hind hoof strikes the back of the front foot or leg; sometimes results in the front shoe being stepped on and pulled off.

P-3. See *coffin bone*.

PIII. See *coffin bone*.

packing. Material used to fill the space between a full pad and the sole of the hoof; keeps dirt from being trapped under the pad. Packing material may contain antibiotics and medications for therapeutic uses and to prevent growth of undesirable microorganisms.

pad. Material cut to the outside shape of the horseshoe and applied between the shoe and hoof.

pastern. The area between the fetlock joint and the hoof.

pastern angle. Angle between the pastern and level ground as seen from the side when the horse is standing square.

periople. Narrow strip below the coronary band that functions somewhat like the human cuticle; produces a waxy protective coating that migrates down the hoof.

plantar. Refers to the sole of the foot.

posterior. Toward or on the rear; opposite of anterior.

preventive trimming and shoeing. Characterized by trimming and shoeing for balance, support, and protection; efforts made to achieve long-term soundness and performance longevity by preventing hoof problems.

proximal. Close to the torso; opposite of distal.

quarter. Portion of the hoof between the heel and the toe.

quarter clip. See *clip*.

quarter crack. See *crack*.

quick. Sensitive laminae between the hoof wall and the coffin bone; or to drive a nail into the sensitive laminae.

resection. Removal of part of an organ or structure; for example, the cutting away of a part of the hoof wall in the case of laminitis.

reset. To remove a horseshoe, trim the hoof, and then reattach the same horseshoe.

rim pad. Pad inserted between the hoof and the shoe that does not cover the sole or frog.

rim shoe. Horseshoe with a deep crease or groove in the ground surface from heel to heel, dividing the shoe into two rims; used for mild traction.

rocker toe. Horseshoe that has been bent upward toward the hoof at the toe; used to ease and direct breakover.

rolled toe. Horseshoe that has been rounded or beveled on the outer edge of the ground surface at the toe; used to ease breakover.

rotation. The movement of the coffin bone within the hoof capsule caused by separation of the laminae, usually as a result of laminitis.

rununder heels. See *underrun heels*.

seedy toe. Stretching and separation of the white line of the hoof, usually at the toe; often a result of chronic laminitis.

sensitive laminae. See *laminae*.

shelly. Refers to a weak hoof wall that tends to split easily and flake away.

short shoeing. Applying a horseshoe that is not long enough to provide adequate support for the foot and leg.

side clip. See *clip*.

sinker. Result of laminitis, when the coffin bone sinks straight down within the hoof without rotating.

sliding plate. Wide, smooth-surfaced horseshoe used on the hind feet of reining horses to facilitate sliding stops.

snowballing. Buildup of snow on the hoof bottom.

sole. The horny covering on the bottom of the hoof between the hoof wall and the frog.

spooned heel. Spooned-heel shoe; a horseshoe that has had the tips of the heels forged thin and bent up to fit closely to the heels of the hoof; used to prevent the heels of the front shoes from being stepped on by the toes of the hind shoes.

sprung shoe. Shoe that is caught or stepped on and bent, yet remains nailed to the hoof.

squared toe. Horseshoe with the toe shaped straight across; usually fit so the toe of the hoof extends over the shoe; used to ease breakover and prevent forging.

tendon. Strong inelastic tissue that connects muscle to bone.

tenotomy. Surgical severing of a tendon.

therapeutic shoeing. Shoeing to protect and support a damaged hoof or limb or to prevent or encourage a particular movement until healing can take place.

thrush. Foul-smelling black exudates of anaerobic bacteria that thrive in the warm, dark recesses of the hoof.

toed in. Conformation defect in which a horse's hoof points inward; horses having both forefeet toed in are called pigeon-toed.

toed out. Conformation defect in which a horse's hoof points outward.

trailer. Extra-long heel on a horseshoe that usually angles away from the centerline of the hoof.

tube pad. Type of rim pad with a hollow tube that fits against the inside edge of the horseshoe; used to prevent snow and dirt from packing into the bottom of the hoof.

tubules. Fibers that make up the bulk of the hoof wall; they run parallel to each other and perpendicular to the coronary band.

underrun heels. Often-irreversible condition in which the angle of the hoof wall at the heels is lower than the toe angle by 5 degrees or more. Also called underslung heels and rununder heels.

underslung heels. See *underrun heels*.

unilateral. On only one side.

unsound. Refers to a horse that has a defect or condition that could lead to lameness; an unsound horse might not be currently lame.

web. Refers to the width of a branch of a horseshoe.

wedge pad. Hoof pad that is thick at one end and tapers to very thin at the other; commonly used to elevate the heels. Also called a degree pad.

wedge shoe. Horseshoe that is thicker in the heels than the toe; used for raising the hoof angle to balance the foot.

white line disease (WLD). Deterioration of the white line caused by invasion of the laminae by bacteria, yeast, or fungus; evidenced by a white cheesy material and hollow air pockets.

wide-web shoe. Horseshoe made from wider bar stock than normal.

wild. Untamed animal that runs free and has no ancestors that were domesticated.

X-ray. An image produced by photographing radiation, which passes through visually opaque matter; used to take pictures of bones. Also called radiograph.

RESOURCE GUIDE

FARRIER & VETERINARY ORGANIZATIONS

American Association of Equine Practitioners (AAEP)
Lexington, Kentucky
859-233-0147
www.aaep.org

American Farrier's Association
Lexington, Kentucky
859-233-7411
www.americanfarriers.org

The Guild of Professional Farriers
Washington, D.C.
www.guildfarriers.org

Brotherhood of Working Farriers Association
LaFayette, Georgia
706-397-8047
www.bwfa.net

INFORMATION

Horsekeeping.com
Hundreds of online articles on hoof care, health care, training, facilities and horse management, and instructions for applying a CVP pad
www.horsekeeping.com

Horseshoes.com
Online forums and over 150,000 pages of farrier, hoof care, and equine health–related material
www.horseshoes.com

Rocky Mountain Research and Consulting, Inc.
Center, Colorado
Current research and prevention of grass founder in horses
www.safergrass.org

Shoeing Rules and Regulations
Provides horse-show regulations from 157 organizations
www.lesspub.com/s3/site/pdf/afj/Shoeing-Rules05.pdf

PRODUCTS

Hoof Sealers/Hardeners

Keratex.net
Brookeville, Maryland
888-537-2839
Hoof sealer, hardener, thrush treatment
www.keratex.net

Glue-On Shoes

Sound Horse Technologies, Inc.
Unionville, Pennsylvania
800-801-2654
Sigafoos Series™
www.soundhorse.com

Hoof Boots

EasyCare, Inc.
Tucson, Arizona
800-447-8836
Easy Boot line, Boa, Old Mac, and Soaker brands
www.easycareinc.com

Plum Shade Farm
Coatesville, Pennsylvania
610-486-0708
HOOFix Emergency Trail Boot and Abscess Kit
www.plumshadefarm.com

Cavallo Horse & Rider
Roberts Creek, British Columbia
877-818-0037
Simple Boot brand
www.cavallo-inc.com/horseboots.html

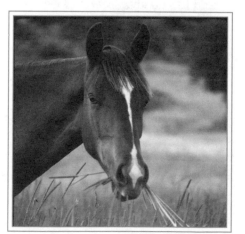

RELATED BOOKS AND VIDEOS BY CHERRY HILL

101 Arena Exercises: A Ringside Guide for Horse and Rider, North Adams, MA: Storey Publishing, 1995.

101 Horsekeeping Tips (DVD), Livermore, CO: Horsekeeping Books and Videos, 2006.

Cherry Hill's Horsekeeping Almanac: The Essential Month-by-Month Guide for Everyone Who Keeps or Cares for Horses, North Adams, MA: Storey Publishing, 2007.

Horse Handling and Grooming, North Adams, MA: Storey Publishing, 1997.

Horse Health Care, North Adams, MA: Storey Publishing, 1997.

Horsekeeping on a Small Acreage: Designing and Managing Your Equine Facilities, Second Edition, North Adams, MA: Storey Publishing, 2005.

How To Think Like A Horse: The Essential Handbook for Understanding Why Horses Do What They Do, North Adams, MA: Storey Publishing, 2006.

Practical Guide to Lameness, Ames, IA: Blackwell Publishing, 2006. By Cherry Hill and Ted Stashak, DVM.

Stablekeeping: A Visual Guide to Safe and Healthy Horsekeeping, North Adams, MA: Storey Publishing, 2000.

INDEX

Pages in *italic* indicate illustrations.

A

abscesses
daily hoof check and, 36
facilities and, 14, 16
treatments for, 13, 44, 60, *60*, 121–22, *121–22*
advertisements for finding a farrier, 12, *12*
"A-frame" stance, 131, *131*
aluminum shoes, 62, *62*, 68
American Association of Equine Practitioners (AAEP), 13
American Farrier's Association (AFA), 12
ammonia, 15, 32
anatomy of horseshoe, 61, *61*
antiseptics for hooves, 6, 43, *43*
applying hoof products, 93–96, *93–96*
asymmetric side clips, 67, *67*
attitude and attention of horse, 115

B

balance
hoof, checking, 49, *49*, 81–82, *81–82*, 118
interfering and, 118
letting horse find his, 87, *87*
movement, shoeing for, 113
balanced diet, 30, *30*, 130, 134
barefoot, 8, 46–56, 97, *97*
"bargain" tack caution, 40
barn (building), site preparation, 14, *14*
bar shoes, 62, *62*
bars of hoof, 2, *2*
bedding, 15, 16, 17, *17*, 32
best shoeing job, staying on the longest (false), 8
black, better than white hooves (false), 6
blacksmiths vs. farriers, 72
black walnut shavings caution, 17
blocking the clinches, 77, *77*
blowouts (horizontal cracks), 103, *103*
boots, 44, *44*, 47, 53–56, *53–56*, 92, *92*, 115, 121
borium for traction, 68, *68*, 70
bottom of hoof, 1–2, *1–2*
branch of horseshoe, 61, *61*
breakover, 50, *50*, 119, *119*, 126, *126*
"broken back" hoof angle, 3, *3*, 82, *82*, 97, *97*
"broken forward" hoof angle, 3, *3*, 82, *82*
broken walls, 5
Brotherhood of Working Farriers Association (BWFA), 12
bruises/bruising, 14, 36, 60, *60*, 120–22, *120–22*
brushes, 42, *42*
brushing hoof wall, 38, *38*
bubble pads, 65, *65*, 70, *70*
bulletin boards for finding a farrier, 12, *12*

C

calks for traction, 67, 68
cannon bone, 3, *3*, *125*
cardboard for floor protection, 94, *94*
central cleft or sulcus, 2, *2*
"certified farrier," 12

chestnut reflex, 25, *25*
clean and dry stalls, 32–33, *32–33*
cleaning hooves, 35, *35*, 38, *38*
clinch/clinches
blocking the, 77, *77*
checking, 85, *85*
closing the, 78, *78*
filing, 78, *78*, 85, *85*, 88, *88*
loose, 37, *37*
opening the, 88, *88*
clinch cutters, 45, *45*
clips, horseshoes, 67, *67*
close nail, showing, 79, *79*
closing the clinches, 78, *78*
clubfoot, 123–24, *123–24*
clutter in work areas caution, 20, *20*
coffin bone, 2, *2*, 3, *3*
fractured, 60
laminitis and, 128, *128–29*, 129, 133, *133*
nail paths and, 79, *79*
navicular syndrome and, 125, *125–26*, 126
coffin bone angle, 3, *3*, 76, *76*, 109, *109*
cold or hot shoes, 72–73, *73*
colic, 16, 17
collateral clefts or sulci, 2, *2*
Colorado State University Veterinary Teaching Hospital, 66
concrete stall flooring, 16
conditioning bare feet, 47, 48, 49
cone shape of hoof, 5, *5*
confidence increased from shoeing, 59, *59*
conformation and interfering, 118
contracted heels, 5, *5*, 109, 112, *112*, 125
corner, avoiding getting trapped in, 87, *87*
corns and veterinary care, 121, *121*
coronary band (coronet), 2, *2*, 4, *4*, 34, *34*, 105
corrective trimming, shoeing, 7, *7*, 51, 52, *52*, 57
costs of shoeing, 10
cotton lead ropes, 40, *40*
cracks. *See* hoof cracks
crease nail cutters, 45, *45*
crease (swedge) of horseshoe, 61, *61*
cross-ties, 21, *21*, 41
CVP (copper sulfate, Venice turpentine, and polypropylene hoof felt), 66, *66*, 122

D

daily hoof check, 34–37, *34–37*
degree (wedge) pads, 65, *65*, 100, *100*
diet, balanced diet, 30, *30*, 130, 134
directories of farriers, 12
dishes and flares, 5, *5*, 75, *75*, 84, *84*
distal phalanx. *See* coffin bone
dogs and farriers, 140, *140*
do-it-yourself trimming and shoeing, 11
domesticated horses, 46, 47, 57
dorsal-palmar (DP) balance, 82, *82*
do's and don'ts, farrier visits, 142
DP (dorsal-palmar) balance, 82, *82*
draining stall flooring, 15, *15–16*, 16
drains in hoof boots, 56
dressings for hooves, 6, 43, *43*, 93, *93*

"dressing" the hoof, 75, *75*, 84
dryness, facilities, 6, *6*, 14, *14–15*, 17, *17–19*, 18, 19, 30, 32, 107

E

early hoof-handling lessons, 22–23, *22–24*
egg bar shoes, 62, *62*, 111, 113, 127, *127*, 129
electric horse walkers for exercise, 31
elevated toe shoe, 124, *124*
emergency boots, 44, *44*, 92, *92*
environmental factors and hoof quality, 1, 4
euthanasia, 129, 132
"evil," shoeing as necessary (false), 8
exercise for healthy hooves
barefoot and, 46, 47, 49
hoof problems and, 112, 114
infrequent exercise and hoof care, 7
laminitis prevention and, 134
management and hoof care, 30, 31, *31*
expansion, checking for, 37, *37*, 84, *84*
extensor tendon, 2, *2*
eyeballing shoe for levelness, 36, *36*

F

facilities and hoof care, 14–21
false tales, 6–8, *6–8*
farrier
finding a farrier, 12, *12*
keeping a good, 140–41, *140–42*
scheduling, 39, *39*, 52, *52*, 97, 114, 139, *139*
skills of, 10–11, *11*, 12
why you need a, 9
working positions, 26, *26*, 29, *29*
feeding (balanced diet), 30, *30*, 130, 134
feral (wild) horses, 46, 47, *47*, 57, 126, *126*
fetlock hyperextension caution, 31
filing clinches, 78, *78*, 85, *85*, 88, *88*
filling the holes (shoeing), 78, *78*
finding a
farrier, 12, *12*
veterinarian, 13
finishing, shoeing, 78, *78*
first phalanx (long pastern bone), 2–3, *3*, 125
fitting and nailing the shoe, 77, *77*
flares and dishes, 5, *5*, 75, *75*, 84, *84*
flexible-cuff glue-on shoes, 64, *64*
flexor tendon, 2, *2*, 125, *125–26*, 126
flooring of stalls, 15–16, *15–16*, 32, *32*
foaling and laminitis, 135, *135*
foals
early hoof-handling lessons, 22–23, *22–24*
steep hoof angle, 123, *123*
trimming, 51–52, *51–52*
"foot" (command), 24, 25
foot flight, 118
footing in exercise area, 31
"foot" vs. "hoof," 1
forehand, traveling heavy on the, 115
foreign objects, checking for, 35–36, *35–36*
forging, 116–17, *116–17*
45 degree ideal angle (false), 6
forward farrier position, front leg forward, 26, *26*

founder, 122, 128, 133, *133. See also* laminitis
four-point trim, 50
free-choice trace-mineralized salt, 30
frog of hoof, 1, 2, *2*
   laminitis and supporting, 133, *133*
   shedding, 35, *35*
   touching ground for blood circulation
     (false), 7
   trimming the, 74, *74*
front feet, lifting, 24–26, *24–26*
front hoof shape, 4, *4–5*, 5
full flat pads, 65, *65*, 66, 110, *110*, 128
full support shoes, 62, *62*, 105, *105*, 113

G

gaiters of hoof boots, 56, *56*
gait problems corrected from shoeing, 59, *59*
"gate potatoes," 31
genetics and hoof quality, 1, 4
glossary, 144–47
glue-on shoes, 64, *64*
good nail, showing, 79, *79*
good work, knowing, 81–88, *81–88*
"graduate farrier," 12
grain, 30, 134, 135, *135*
grass cracks, 103, 104, *104*
grazing and laminitis, 130, *130*, 134, *134*
ground manners, 22–25, *22–25*, 138, *138*
ground surfaces of horseshoes, 61, *61*
growth and shape of hoof, 4–5, *4–5*
Guild of Professional Farriers (GPF), 12

H

half shoe (tip shoe), 124, *124*
halter classes and hoof polish, 95
halters, 40, 41, *41*
hammers, 45, *45*
hardeners for hooves, 43, *43*, 93, *93*
hardwood wood products for bedding, 17
hay, 30, 134
head movement of horse and balance, 114
head of horse, controlling, 86, *86*
heart bar shoes, 62, *62*, 128, 133, *133*
heel bulbs, 2, *2*, 43, 93, *93*
heel of horseshoe, 61, *61*
heels of hoof, 1, 2
   contracted heels, 5, *5*, 109, 112, *112*, 125
   length and support, checking, 83, *83*
   soreness, 109, 125
   underrun heels, 10, 60, 65, 111, *111*
high/low (mismatched) hooves, 113, *113*
high-rise boot, 54, *54*
"high spots," 73, *73*
hind feet, lifting, 27–29, *27–29*
hind hoof shape, 4, *4–5*, 5
hock, 3, *3*
holding horse for farrier, 86–87, *86–87*
holes, filling the (shoeing), 78, *78*
hoof and pastern angle
   examples of, 3, *3*, 48, *48*, 82, *82*
   hoof problems and, 97, *97*, 109, *109*
hoof antiseptics, 6, 43, *43*
hoof boots, 44, *44*, 47, 53–56, *53–56*, 92, *92*,
   115, 121
hoof care
   barefoot, 8, 46–56, 97, *97*
   facilities and, 14–21
   hoof knowledge, 1–8

horseshoes, and why, 57–71
   management for, 30–39
   owner skills and, 81–96
   problems and fixes, 97–119
   professional helpers for, 9–13
   shoeing, and how, 72–80
   tack and tools, 40–45
   teamwork for, 13, 136–42
   training and, 22–29
   veterinary care, 13, *13*, 35, 120–35,
     138, *138*
hoof care hokum, 6–8, *6–8*
hoof cracks, 103–6
   causes of, 5, 6, 14, 33, 109
   daily hoof check and, 33, 34, *34*
   treatments for, 10, 13, 105–6, *105–6*
   types of, 103–4, *103–4*
hoof dressings, 6, 43, *43*, 93, *93*
hoof gauge (protractor), 76, *76*
hoof hardeners, 43, *43*, 93, *93*
hoof horn, 2, *2*
hoof packing, 66, *66*, 122, 128, 129
hoof polishes, 6, 43, *43*, 95–96, *95–96*
hoof products, applying, 93–96, *93–96*
hoof sealers, 43, *43*, 94, *94*, 106
hoof stand, 26, 29, 42, *42*
hoof testers, 125, 131, 138
hoof wall, 2, *2*, 38, *38*, 79, *79*
horizontal cracks (blowouts), 103, *103*
horseshoe nail, 79, *79*
horseshoes, and why, 57–71. *See also* shoeing,
   and how
hot nail, 13, 79, *79*
hot or cold shoes, 72–73, *73*
human hand and horse foot comparison, 3, *3*

I

ice nails for traction, 68, *68*
imbalance, 49, *49*, 113
insensitive hoof tissues, 1, 2, 79, *79*
inside a hoof, 2, *2*
interfering, 7, 118–19, *118–19*
interlocking rubber mats, 16, *16*

K

keeping a good farrier, *140–41*, 140–42
keg shoes, 61
kids and farriers, 140
knee of horse, 3, *3*
knock-kneed foals, 51, *51*
knowing good work when you see it, 81–88,
   81–88

L

lameness, 13, 14, 31, 36, 47, 79, 104, 122, 125
laminae, 2, *2*, 128, *128–29*, 129
laminitis, 9, 10, 17, 60, 128–35, *128–35*
lead ropes, 40, *40*
learning by farriers, 11, *11*
length (excess) and broken hooves, 49, *49*
levelness of shoe, 36, *36*
longeing for exercise, 31, *31*
long pastern bone, *2–3*, 3, 125
long-toe/low-heel (LT/LH), 109–11
   balance and, 82
   breakover and, 50
   hoof problems and, 109–11, *109–11*,
    112, 115

   lengthening stride from (false), 6
   navicular syndrome and, 125
   seedy toe and, 122
loose clinch, 37, *37*
loose nail head, 36, *36*
lost shoes, 5, 98–102, *98–102*
low rider boot, 54, *54*
LT/LH. *See* long-toe/low-heel

M

management and hoof care, 30–39
maneuvering, leaving room for, 87, *87*
mats, stall flooring, 15, *15–16*, 16
mattress for stall, waterproof, 16
measuring and balancing the hoof, 76, *76*
medial-lateral (ML) balance, 81, *81*
medical support from shoeing, 60, *60*
mild steel for horseshoes, 61
mismatched (high/low) hooves, 113, *113*
ML (medial-lateral) balance, 81, *81*
modified-toe shoes, 63, *63*, 111
moist hoofprint, 66
mud, 6, *6*, 8, 33, *33*, 98, *98*
mustang roll, 50, *50*
muzzle for grazing, 134, *134*

N

nail head, loose, 36, *36*
nail holes of horseshoe, 61, *61*
nailing the shoe, 77, *77*
nail/nails
   horseshoe, 79, *79*
   pattern and clinches, checking, 85, *85*
   pulling each individually, 89, *89*
   removing from hoof, 90, *90*
natural-balance trim, 50
natural materials for stall flooring, 15–16,
   15–16
natural trim, 50
navicular bone, 2, *2*
navicular syndrome, 125–27, *125–27*
   hoof problems and, 97, 109, 115
   professional help with, 9, 10
   treatments for, 60, 65, 127, *127*
neglected hooves, 97, *97*, 114
new shoes or reset, 80, *80*
nipping the wall, 74, *74*
noseband of halter, fitting, 41, *41*
nutrition (balanced diet), 30, *30*, 130, 134
nylon lead ropes, 40, *40*
nylon web halters, 41, *41*

O

"off," 123
opening the clinches, 88, *88*
opposite shoe, stepping on, 100, *100*
out in the open, holding horse for farrier,
   86, *86*
overreaching, 99, *99*, 116–17, *116–17*
owner
   role as team captain, 137–38, *137–38*
   skills and hoof care, 81–96
   working positions, 26, *26*, 28, *28*

P

P1 (long pastern bone), *2–3*, 3, 125
P2 (short pastern bone), *2–3*, 3, 125
P3/PIII. *See* coffin bone

packing (hoof), 66, *66*, 122, 128, 129
"paddling," 7
pads, 65, *65*, 66, 70, *70*, 110, *110*, 128
parts of hoof and function, 1–2, *1–2*
pastern. *See* hoof and pastern angle
pasture and pens, 18–19, *18–19*, 30
pasture trim, 50
pawing, imbalance from, 49, *49*
pedal bone. *See* coffin bone
pens and pasture, 18–19, *18–19*, 30
percolation rate of soil, testing, 14
periople, 2, *2*, 4, *4*, 93
physical problems and stumbling, 115
picking out hooves, 35, *35*, 38, *38*
picking up the feet, 24–25, *24–25*
picks, 42, *42*
pigeon-toed (pointing in), 7, *7*, 52, *52*
pivot point, 50, *50*, 63, 127
placenta (retained) and laminitis, 135, *135*
plain horseshoes, 61, *61*, 68, 128
pointing in (pigeon-toed), 7, *7*, 52, *52*
pointing out (splay-footed), 7, *7*
pointing straight ahead, hooves (false), 7, *7*
polishes for hooves, 6, 43, *43*, 95–96, *95–96*
ponying for exercise, 31
preventative hoof care, 57
problems and fixes, 97–119
products for hooves, 43, *43*, 93–96, *93–96*
professional helpers, 9–13
protection for hoof, temporary, 91–92, *91–92*
protractor (hoof gauge), 76, *76*
prying the heel of the nail, 89, *89*
pulling a shoe, whose job is it?, 13. *See also*
    removing a shoe
pulling each nail individually, 89, *89*
pull-offs, 45, *45*, 89, *89–90*, 90
pulse (horse's), checking, 131, *131*, 135, *135*

Q
quarter clips, 67, *67*
quarter-crack treatment, 105, *105*
quarters of hoof, 1, 2
questions, asking farrier, 85
"quicking" a horse, 79

R
rasping the hoof, 75, *75*
rasps, 45, *45*
reasons for shoeing, 58–60, *58–60*
recommendations for finding a farrier, 12
removing a shoe
    hoof problems and, 101
    pulling a shoe, whose job is it?, 13
    shoe removal kit, 45, *45*
    steps of, 88–90, *88–90*
    winter and, 48, *48*, 69
resetting shoes, 37, *37*, 80, *80*, 101, *101*
resources, 148–49
retain placenta and laminitis, 135, *135*
riding boots, 44, *44*, 53, *53*
riding for exercise, 31
rim pads, 65, *65*
rim shoes, 61, *61*, 68
rocker-toe shoes, 63, *63*
rolled-toe shoes, 63, *63*
rope halters, 41, *41*
rope walking, 115

S
safety, 26–29, *26–29*, 40, 87, *87*
sand bedding, 17
sand colic, 16
sand cracks, 104, *104*
"saw horse" stance, 131, *131*
scheduling farrier, 39, *39*, 52, *52*, 97, 114,
    139, *139*
sealers for hooves, 43, *43*, 94, *94*, 106
second phalanx (short pastern bone), 2–3,
    3, *125*
seedy toe, 5, 122
sensitive hoof tissues, 1, 2, 79, *79*
shaping the foot, 75, *75*
shedding frog, 35, *35*
sheet bend knot, 41, *41*
shifted shoe, resetting, 101, *101*
shod hoof, neglected, 97, *97*
shoeing, and how, 72–80. *See also* horseshoes,
    and why
shoeing areas, 20–21, *20–21*
shoe removal kit, 45, *45*
short pastern bone, 2–3, *3*, 125
short shoeing, 83, *83*, 99
showing, rules, 65, 95, 96, *96*
shredded paper for bedding, 17
side clips, 67, *67*
side-to-side balance, 81, *81*
silent partner, horse as, 136, *136*
site preparation for building a barn, 14, *14*
skills of farriers, 10–11, *11*, 12
sliding plates, 59, *59*, 63, *63*
snaps on lead ropes, 40, *40*
snowballing, 69, *69*, 70
sole of hoof, 1, 2, *2*
    protecting a sensitive, 91, *91*
    trimming the, 74, *74*
solid rubber mats, stall flooring, 16, *16*
solid stall flooring, 15, *15*
splay-footed (pointing out), 7, *7*
spooned-heel shoe, 100, *100*
sprung shoe, 101, *101*
squared toe shoes, 62, *62–63*, 63, 99, *99*, 105,
    111, 113, 117, *117*, 127, *127*
stalls and pens, 15–16, *15–16*, 32–33, *32–33*
stamped shoes, 61, *61*
steel horseshoes, 61
stepped off shoes, 98–102, *98–102*
stone, lodged under heels of shoe, 36, *36*
straight bar shoes, 62, *62*, 127, *127*
stratum tectorum, 2, *2*, 4, *4*, 93
straw bedding, 17
studs for traction, 55, *55*, 68, *68*
stumbling, 114–15, 125
sugar and laminitis, 130, *130*, 134, *134*
Sugardine, 107, 108, *108*
sulci, 2, *2*
supplements, 30
support provided from shoeing, 58, *58*
surface cracks, 103, *103*
swedge (crease) of horseshoe, 61, *61*
swiveled shoe, 101, *101*
synthetic shoes, 64, *64*

T
tab glue-on shoes, 64, *64*
tack and tools, 40–45
tack (ill-fitting) and stumbling, 115

tape for temporary hoof protection, 91, *91*
teamwork for hoof care, 13, 136–42
temporary hoof protection, 91–92, *91–92*
tendon reflex, 25, *25*
tenotomy, 124
therapeutic shoeing, 57
third phalanx. *See* coffin bone
thrush, 14, 97, 106, 107–8, *107–8*
time of farrier, valuable, 10, *10*
tip shoe (half shoe), 124, *124*
toe clips, 67, *67*
toed-out hinds, 119, *119*
toe of hoof, 1, 2
    cracks, 105, *105–6*, 106
    length, measuring, 76, *76*
toe of horseshoe, 61, *61*
tools, 42, *42*
toughening bare feet, 47, 48, 49
traction, 55, *55*, 58, *58*, 61, 65, 67, 68, *68*,
    69, 70
training and hoof care, 22–29
treadmills for exercise, 31
treatment boots, 44, *44*
treatment-plate shoes, 60, *60*, 121
trimming, 49–52, *49–52*, 74, *74*
tube-type rim pads, 65, *65*, 70, *70*
twisting off nail ends, 77, *77*
tying options, 21, *21*

U
underrun heels, 10, 60, 65, 111, *111*

V
vanity shoeing, 57
veterinary care, 13, *13*, 35, 120–35, 138, *138*
vital signs, knowing normal, 131

W
walkers (electric) for exercise, 31
wall, holding horse for farrier, 87, *87*
wall of hoof, 1, 2
water
    applying before hoof dressing, 93
    standing in for soft hooves (false), 6, *6*
waterproof stall mattress, 16
wear (excessive) prevention from shoeing,
    58, *58*
wear of shoe, 80, *80*
web halters, 41, *41*
wedge (degree) pads, 65, *65*, 100, *100*
weight, maintaining healthy, 30
white hooves, black, better than (false), 6
white line, 2, *2*
white line disease (WLD), 14, 122, *122*
wide web shoes, 62, *62*
wild (feral) horses, 46, 47, *47*, 57, 126, *126*
window resection for laminitis, 133, *133*
"winging out," 7
winter and shoeing, 48, *48*, 58, *58*, 69–70,
    69–71
WLD (white line disease), 14, 122, *122*
wood products for bedding, 17, *17*
wood stall flooring, 16
work areas, 20–21, *20–21*
working positions, 26–29, *26–29*

OTHER STOREY TITLES YOU WILL ENJOY

Cherry Hill's Horsekeeping Skills Library.
A wealth of practical advice on developing essential skills to maintain consistent equine well-being, from an award-winning horse handler. Latest title is *Horse Hoof Care*. Other titles in the series are *Horse Handling & Grooming, Horse Health Care, Stablekeeping,* and *Trailering Your Horse.* Paper. Learn more about each title by visiting *www.storey.com.*

Cherry Hill's Horsekeeping Almanac.
The essential month-by-month guide to establishing good routines and following natural cycles to be the best horsekeeper you can be. 576 pages. Paper. ISBN 978-1-58017-684-2.

The Foaling Primer, by Cynthia McFarland.
A chronicle of the first year of a horse's life in amazing, up-close photographs and detailed descriptions. 160 pages. Paper. ISBN 978-1-58017-608-8.

The Horse Conformation Handbook, by Heather Smith Thomas.
A detailed "tour of the horse," analyzing all aspects of conformation and discussing how variations will affect a horse's performance. 400 pages. Paper. ISBN 978-1-58017-558-6.

Horsekeeping on a Small Acreage, by Cherry Hill.
A thoroughly updated, full-color edition of the author's best-selling classic about how to have efficient operations and happy horses. 320 pages. Paper. ISBN 978-1-58017-535-7. Hardcover. ISBN 978-1-58017-603-3.

How to Think Like a Horse, by Cherry Hill.
Detailed discussions of how horses think, learn, respond to stimuli, and interpret human behavior — in short, a light on the equine mind. 192 pages. Paper. ISBN 978-1-58017-835-8. Hardcover. ISBN 978-1-58017-836-5.

Stable Smarts, by Heather Smith Thomas.
A treasure-trove of equine know-how, assembled by an Idaho horsewoman, for riders and owners everywhere. 320 pages. Paper. ISBN 978-1-58017-610-1.

Storey's Horse-Lover's Encyclopedia, edited by Deborah Burns.
A user-friendly, A-to-Z guide to all things equine that includes line drawings, lists, diagrams, and helpful tips. 484 pages. Paper. ISBN 978-1-58017-317-9.